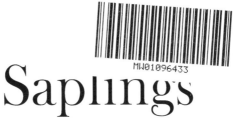

Saplings
On the Path to Mastery in
Acupuncture and Herbal Medicine

Edited by

Carl Stimson

Visit the book's website at www.saplingsbook.com

Printed in the United States of America

First Printing: June 2012

ISBN-13: 978-0615626550

Publisher:

Carl Stimson
6123 Moondance Rd.
Helena, MT 59601
carlstimson@gmail.com

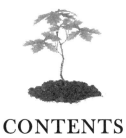

CONTENTS

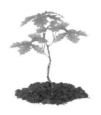

INTRODUCTION
BY CARL STIMSON

My education in acupuncture and herbal medicine took three years; eight semesters, to be exact. In my last semester I took a series of relatively simple written tests from a national accreditation organization, then was granted the status of "Diplomate of Oriental Medicine." This, along with my diploma, made me eligible for an acupuncture license in most of the fifty U.S. states. After jumping through various bureaucratic hoops to obtain licenses first in Montana and then in Massachusetts, I was free to practice much as I saw fit – there was no supervised postgraduate internship.

Practitioners of Oriental medicine[1] in Western nations that do not have draconian regulations, which is most of them, have vast freedom in choosing what to do with their newly licensed skills. Success is difficult to achieve, but the opportunities to try are virtually unrestricted. This field outside of Asia is young, although it has put down some substantial roots recently, and this youth means the landscape is wide open and ready to be shaped. There is a huge untapped population of potential patients who have never experienced acupuncture or herbal medicine, and practitioners have yet to discover how these people can best be reached. Parts of this field that are currently large and influential, such as community acupuncture and cosmetic needling, barely had a presence when I entered school in 2004. I have no doubt that other major transformations are to come.

While there is great freedom to create and succeed, the risk of failure is perhaps greater. Graduates leave school with extensive knowledge of points and plants, but only a sprinkling of business education, conse-

---

[1] Oriental medicine includes massage, qi gong and several other modalities, but here I refer to primarily acupuncture and Asian styles of herbal medicine. Other chapters use the terms Chinese medicine or traditional Chinese medicine (TCM).

quently entering their practices weighed down with fear about their chances for success. There are few secure jobs for acupuncture graduates, forcing most into small-business ownership. Surveys have shown it is not easy: a significant proportion of people with degrees in Oriental medicine are not active in the field five years after graduation, and many others return to the jobs they held before entering school, only needling part-time.

This book contains the stories of sixteen practitioners of Oriental medicine in these dizzy first few years of practice. The title *Saplings* comes from the wood phase of the ancient Chinese concept of the five phases. These stages of transformation (wood, fire, earth, metal, water) are different from the Greek humors in that they do not represent actual substances, but describe the changes and characteristics of natural phenomena – a constant cycle of growth and decay. I find it easier to conceptualize this through the phases' seasonal correspondences (wood = spring, fire = summer, earth = harvest, metal = autumn, water = winter). Wood-spring is the time of birth and rapid growth, but also a time when living things are still immature. Thus the wood phase fits well with the career stage this book describes. A sprout is the type of plant life most often associated with the wood phase, but this as a description of newly minted acupuncturists and herbalists seems too infantile. Practitioners just out of school have, after all, three-plus years of education and hundreds of hours of clinical experience. A sapling, which is young, but with roots strong enough to give it some stability, is a more appropriate representation.

The first steps in any endeavor are likely to be rocky, but by the time one reaches a certain level of competency, memories of this period become hazy or glazed over with nostalgia, like an adult looking back on the teen years. The short time I have treated patients outside my university's intern clinic has been a period of fascinating experiences and radical transformations in how I feel about Oriental medicine. During this time I have completely revamped my technique, gone through enormous changes in my opinions toward numerous aspects of the field, and have been forced to face up to significant weaknesses. Thankfully I have not been alone. Conversations about this process with fellow practitioners has not only helped me regain my stability after being humbled, but has lent this time a curiosity and sense of liberation that were absent in the prescribed curriculum and routine of school.

This feeling of being understood, either by telling someone about your life and knowing the listener really understands, or by realizing someone else's life has led to insights similar to your own, is perhaps one of the most fulfilling experiences there is. This fellowship can be as casual as a conversation with a stranger about the baseball team you both follow or as intimate as a marriage of forty years, and such sharing is an essential part of a fulfilling career.

I studied acupuncture and herbal medicine at a small, family-like school in Honolulu, Hawai'i. The student body was never much larger than thirty people and most classes comprised several grade levels, even sometimes the whole school. In addition to classrooms, the main building included five dorm rooms and a small communal kitchen. This familial setting strengthened the sense of community, as did the large proportion of students who came from the mainland United States to attend school on the remote Pacific island. After graduation, my sense of community with like-minded peers was primarily obtained through one-on-one relationships. There were some good friends I could talk with about anything, from the pros and cons of trigger-point needling to personal family issues; and there were coworkers and acquaintance practitioners with whom I mainly talked shop.

Even back in school, however, I was finding this sense of connection in avenues other than through human contact. I was finding it in books. One book I read early in school that exemplifies this connection is *Acupuncture in Practice: Case History Insights from the West*. Unlike translations of case studies from China, which, when not dry and academic, come with cultural and linguistic gaps that many Westerners have trouble bridging, the patient histories in *Acupuncture in Practice* were story-like, with intimate personal details and anecdotes sitting alongside lab tests and point prescriptions. This was my first glimpse into the shared pool of emotions and experiences of practitioners of Oriental medicine. Bob Flaws' early book *Timing and the Times* showed me that even in a field where the basic tenets were laid down at least 2,000 years ago, there is still a place for exploration, imagination and speculation. Other books I connected to included *Classical Japanese Acupuncture* by Shudo Denmei and *Traditional Acupuncture: Traditional Diagnosis* by J.R. Worsley. Even though I have never practiced the techniques these texts endorse, Meridian Therapy and Five-Element Acupuncture, respectively, I was inspired by the sense of personal journey they conveyed. After graduation Lisa Rohleder's community-acupuncture manifesto *The Remedy* was added to this list.

These reads expanded my understanding of Oriental medicine more deeply than the encyclopedic herbal and point texts that filled my classroom hours. Through them I realized the deeply personal nature of my new career; how treating patients challenges and changes people, and how one must be simultaneously a skilled craftsman, creative artist and consummate communicator. I looked for more writings that addressed these deeper aspects of practice, but quickly saw that Oriental medicine has a dearth of such books. There is a wealth of good and useful texts – herbal and point compendiums, books on specific diseases or body systems, and case history collections. However, in very few do the authors describe the influence of their personal characteristics and circumstances on their professional paths. There is a distinct lack of "I" in the literature, and seeking to make a home in my new field, I wished others had taken more time to describe how they found theirs.

I eventually discovered that biomedical doctors have penned many such books and I began reading them, not to figure out how to use their methods to cure disease, but to dig deeper into what it meant to be a medical practitioner. Though it did not occur to me at the time, this now strikes me as ironic. Many people choose a career in Oriental medicine because of a perceived lack of heart in conventional medicine, but when I sought out insights on the more personal and nebulous side of seeing patients, I was forced to look to the M.D.'s.

Eventually I decided to do something about this vacuity in the literature of the field. But with a career only several years old, I was not about to write a lengthy memoir on my medical journey. Nevertheless, I knew I possessed something valuable that people who have been practicing for thirty years lack: still-fresh intimate knowledge of inexperience. As my story is not yet rich enough to fill a volume on its own, I asked friends and colleagues I knew from school, or had met while practicing and in my travels, to contribute an essay describing what they went through while transforming from a green new graduate into a polished professional.

The sixteen authors in the pages that follow are a diverse group and their stories well represent the opportunities and struggles that are part of this career stage. About one-third of the authors are not U.S. citizens, nearly half were living outside the United States at the time of writing, and the male-female split is nearly even. The only significant bias I see is that eight of the authors attended the same small school as myself in Hawai'i.

As a group, who are these people and what common challenges and dreams have shaped them? Before receiving any draft chapters, I knew in some sense what to expect – after all, I belong to this crowd – but what I did not expect was the nuanced and varied ways these themes would be expressed. Readers who are themselves green practitioners will find much to identify with in the chapters to come. More seasoned practitioners will no doubt see many of their early experiences reflected in the authors' stories, but will also see that this generation of practitioners enters a very different environment. For example, some things that were nonexistent in the field's early days in the West, such as licensure, the possibility of insurance compensation and easy access to the tools of the trade, are now taken for granted.

It is my experience that most people see Oriental medicine as a foreign and unusual career choice. While a retail shop owner and an engineer may share little in the way of education or job experience, both likely have a rough understanding of what the other's career entails in terms of education and day-to-day routine. When encountering practitioners of Oriental medicine, however, people have difficulty making such a connection. When I say I am an acupuncturist, I can almost see them asking themselves, "What kind of person would choose such a [weird/fascinating] career?" Most non-acupuncturists who have chosen to pick up this book would likely choose "fascinating" over "weird," but this sense of distance remains. In the chapters that follow, it will become clear that while practitioners of Oriental medicine have indeed made a unique career choice, they share many struggles and joys with people in other careers.

Acupuncture has been known outside Asia for centuries, but the field only started to flourish in the West in the 1970s, when the first acupuncture schools were founded and some U.S. states began licensing practitioners. The profession is now well-established in most Western countries – with official licensing, government loans available for study, limited insurance coverage, and not insignificant recognition by the public and media of acupuncture's therapeutic value – but is not what I would call mature.

This growing acceptance and professionalism have had a significant impact on the type of person who practices acupuncture. Thirty-plus years ago, you could lump practitioners of Oriental medicine in the

West into two broad categories – hippies and native Asians. Immigrants, mostly from China but also Korea and Japan, opened clinics in their adopted homes, but their spheres of influence were often limited to their own communities, usually Chinatowns in major cities. The group that did much of the heavy lifting in the early stages of bringing Oriental medicine in from the fringes was the alternative crowd. For a long time, the path to an acupuncture career for a U.S. or European native very often led through the counterculture movement, such as via an initial interest in Buddhism or macrobiotic eating.

This is changing as Oriental medicine becomes more mainstream. In schools one can now encounter nurses frustrated with Western medicine's limitations or just wanting to expand their skill set, young people who were treated with acupuncture or herbs as children and were inspired to make a career of it, and sharp entrepreneurs hoping to make a buck off the growing popularity of alternative medicine. Most students come from middle-class backgrounds and already have a university degree when they start studying Oriental medicine. Still, alternative interests and lifestyles are much more prevalent in acupuncture schools than in the general public. But while the schools are becoming more representative, society is becoming more accepting of alternative lifestyles. After all, practicing meditation or eating organic food no longer raises many eyebrows, especially in big cities. When I tell someone I am an acupuncturist, the most common reaction is, "Cool!"

Nevertheless, the old guard of (ex-)hippies and native Asians still holds considerable sway over the field. They own the publishing and herb companies, they write the texts and select which books will be translated, and run both the schools and professional organizations. Although one can (and people do) debate the merits and demerits of what the field's founders have done and how they did it, this is not the venue for such a discussion. However, the face of our profession is changing and I feel very strongly that its new voice is worth listening to. I thank Rebecca Parker for expressing this sentiment so eloquently in the preface.

One major issue nearly all acupuncturists and herbalists deal with is the tension between a Western upbringing and the Eastern mode of thought they have chosen to study. The issue is approached in different ways, with one edge of the spectrum being full immersion in the language and culture of the East (as described by Suzanne Robidoux and Emily Smith) and the other end a rejection of classical Chinese thought in favor of modern scientific concepts (as David Vitello talks about). Most practitioners attempt to find ways for the two to coexist and, if possible, supplement each other (see parts of John Renna's essay). Although the chapters just mentioned most directly address the East-West dichotomy, this theme is present in nearly all the essays, though sometimes beneath the surface. Personally, in the seven years since I started studying Oriental medicine, I have gone back and forth on this continuum, constantly moving toward or away from the precision of modern science and the wide sweeps of Oriental medical theory in what sometimes seems like a love-hate relationship.

Another major theme evident in the book is how people come to terms with the business side of the profession. Ask an acupuncturist how he or she chose this occupation as a career, and you will likely hear about being inspired by an experience or book, or wanting to deepen a commitment to certain values, although more practical reasons such as finding a stable career or supporting a family have become more common. Many students get swept up in the beauty and power of Oriental medicine, thrilled to be learning about the mysteries of the body and how to help people. But thoughts about how one will make a living with an acupuncture degree often sit uncomfortably unaddressed in the back of one's mind, like the proverbial elephant in the room.

Schools do an adequate job of educating students how in to needle and prescribe herbs, but practice management and business classes form only a sliver of the curriculum, and are often of quite poor quality. In this collection, not one author expresses misgivings about a lack of academic knowledge, but nearly every entry touches on the trials and tribulations of growing a practice (most directly addressed by Ian Stones and Tara Mattes).

While everyone must surmount business hurdles, patient relations and communication also are prominent concerns in the first years of practice. New acupuncturists do not leave school completely green, as each college runs an intern clinic that offers low-priced treatments from more advanced students. People who frequent these clinics understand they are guinea pigs in the education of acupuncturists and herbalists, and they relax their standards and expectations accordingly. They allow the interns who treat them to indulge in extensive questioning and physical exams during intakes, and wait patiently while the interns confer with supervisors over their conditions. This drawn-out questioning and conferring, as well as a tendency to experiment with methods recently learned in the classroom, make for very practitioner-centered treatments. Not that the goal of healing the patient is ignored, but the intern's education plays a major role in the narrative.

Entering professional practice, however, new practitioners must learn how to make the treatment process primarily patient-centered. Self-indulgent habits from the intern clinic need to be abandoned, and the tolerance bought with the student clinic's low price tag evaporates. Understanding patients' needs and finding ways to address them efficiently and effectively are suddenly matters of life and death, taking precedence over needling skills and diagnostics, which became relatively polished during school. In the chapters that follow, many of the authors discuss not how they *treat* patients, but how they *relate* to patients. Practitioners in the first years of practice often adjust their needling techniques, but it seems that they are more often challenged over issues regarding patient care.

The path of development is nevertheless far from standard, and a final thing that is evident when reading the authors' stories is the individuality and variety of what people do after graduation. People who choose to study Oriental medicine are, if nothing else, a unique lot, but as students are actually quite homogeneous. The routine and requirements of school are relatively confining, with the avenues of practice limited to the intern clinic and possibly an externship organized by the school, and the theories available for exploration largely circumscribed by the curriculum. When I was in school, it seemed like the only thing to do after licensure was start a practice and begin needling. Life, it turns out, is not so simple. After graduation people set off on vastly different journeys, doing different things at different times and in different ways, with each avenue entailing particular joys and worries.

Many of the contributors naturally started their own practices or found work under another practitioner after graduation. There are two, however, who went to China and saw their lives take drastic turns. Two people obtained additional degrees in Oriental medicine (one in California and the other in Japan). Another two chose to return to school to study subjects that built on their medical foundation (public health, nursing), and the contributors who founded community clinics learned of the community-acupuncture business model late in their school careers. There are many other examples of how people chose to deviate from the standard school-license-practice route, or how life chose deviations for them.

I find these differences inspiring and even if the story was written by someone I have never met or about something I have never done, they were all easy to relate to. Myself and the other authors spent three-plus years immersed in Oriental medicine, and it has soaked in deeply. When that background is encountered in others, no matter how different the external manifestations, an affinity springs up, like meeting someone from one's hometown in a far-away land.

This feeling of unity combined with the diverse individuality is what I see as the book's greatest strength.

The contributors chose to tell their stories in a wide variety of ways. Some focus on specific issues or experiences, others capture the feeling of being a green practitioner in broad strokes. Some essays involve limited periods of weeks or months, while others are journeys that span years or decades. Each tale on its own gives a unique glimpse into a thoughtful person's view on their budding career, but when taken together the essays are a snapshot of this special field at a moment when it also is growing from childhood into maturity.

So, without further ado, I hope you will enjoy reading the experiences of this group of acupuncturists and herbalists as they strive to grow tall and put down deep roots in the field of Oriental medicine.

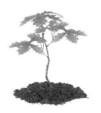

PREFACE: THE NEW BREED
BY REBECCA PARKER

There is a new generation of East Asian medicine practitioners in the West. We are young and smart, and could have gone to medical school if that was how we thought we could have helped the most. We think there is a place in the mainstream for the techniques we have learned, and not just as an "alternative." Although it may have played a part, we did not get into this out of a fascination with Chinese culture, or a desire to escape our own communities, or a hope of being healed ourselves. We see our knowledge and skills as a way to fill the gaps in the narrative of health and disease that we have inherited in our twenty-first century Western culture, and as a part of the search for knowledge and truth about relieving suffering. Our capable minds are curious and nimble enough to embrace the contradictions of Eastern and Western thought. We are interested in the science as well as the art of East Asian medicine, and look forward to a day when it will be called just... medicine.

We are coming into our own in an era when most people we meet have at least heard of acupuncture, and have heard it might be able to help things like weight loss, quitting smoking or back pain. But most people we meet do not know what qi is, or else equate it with something out of reach or weird, somewhere on the woo-woo scale between yoga and crystals. They could not care less about balancing their yin and yang, but would like to increase circulation, regulate their central nervous system, and encourage homeostasis or better yet, allostasis - the maintenance of stability amid constantly shifting conditions.

There will be a need for thinkers like us who can build bridges between the old and the new, between different ways of thinking, between a medicine grounded in fixed anatomical ideas and one based on fluid functional concepts. We face a world where the limits of Western medicine are being met. MRSA presents a challenge that could be over-come by using berberine-containing herbs that cause antibiotics to re-gain their potency against previously resistant bacteria. Concepts such as "sticky blood" are showing up in Western medicine, echoing the thousands-year-old idea of blood stagnation. Research that validates the mind-body connection is coming to light in subjects such as the enteric nervous system and psychoneuroimmunology. These are exciting times.

We bring passion for seeing the changes in our patients, for improv-ing lives, for making the world better in small or not-so-small ways. As we move forward on our paths toward individual and collective mas-tery, and in addition to our daily clinical challenges, we face the ques-tions of how to make this medicine more accessible, how to create a structure for employing new graduates, how to integrate Western and Eastern medical thought, and how not to repeat the mistakes of the American health-care system. We are stronger when we do not just dis-appear into our treatment rooms, but when we encourage each other to be ambitious, to think big, and envision the best for ourselves and all people who need relief from suffering. We have a lot of work to do.

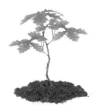

SWIMMING IN THE DAO
BY TARA MATTES

I want to begin my reflection with gratitude. I feel so fortunate to have a path that nourishes and inspires me. What started out as a career interest has evolved into a way of life. Traditional Chinese medicine (TCM) provides a rich framework for comprehending experience, and its Daoist roots give depth and grounding. I continually lean on it as I attempt to understand my own experience and those of others. I am forever thankful to have TCM as a reference and guide to daily living. It has changed the way I look at the world, and hence changed my world. I have found, over the years, that as I help others, I help myself. As I find more compassion for others, I find more for myself. As I encourage others to breathe from their abdomen, I am reminding myself. When I needle Yin Tang, my own furrowed brow relaxes. Going to work has become a form of active meditation and I am thankful everyday for it.

I began my journey into acupuncture as a patient of a very talented and painful Taiwanese acupuncturist. Although it always proved to be a somewhat frightening experience, the results were remarkable and kept me coming back. During this time I had just returned to school to fulfill the prerequisites for becoming a physician's assistant. I started working in a community health clinic and although I loved helping people, I found the actual medicine was not my interest. I had never really thought about a career in acupuncture. I guess, I figured I was not Asian enough. In fact I was not Asian at all and I had never met an acupuncturist that was not. But as my current track seemed to be leading me down a path that no longer felt right to me, I took a chance on what did feel right, and a year later I landed in Hawai'i and enrolled in acupuncture college.

What started out as a daunting four-year commitment soon felt like not enough time. The first three years were a balancing act of work and school; the last year a tightrope of school, a newborn baby and single motherhood. Finishing my degree seemed like a race, a battle and often a fog. There were many sleepless nights when I doubted my ability to finish. Somehow, I just kept moving forward, but in the end I miraculously passed my exams and finished the last remaining treatments to complete my internship. Since I used every available minute to complete school, preparation for my own clinic was seriously neglected. Nonetheless, the world was at my doorstep whether I was ready or not.

One day during those last few weeks, I took a breath, leaned back on the couch and thought, "I have no time to open my own business. I need a job. I need to work for someone like Dr. L." Dr. L was a naturopath I had met while looking for a midwife, and I had instantly been drawn to her energy, work and vision. I ended up moving temporarily to have my baby, so I did not have her as my midwife, but her impression remained. Feeling desperate, I reached for the phone and dialed her number. I got her voice mail and I left an awkward message, "Um… I don't know if you remember me, but, um… My name is Tara Mattes and I'm graduating from acupuncture school… I have experience with birth and um… I was wondering if you needed any help…" I hung up horrified. Did I really just *call* someone for a job? Seriously, not even a resume? I was doomed.

So when the phone rang a week later and Dr. L was on the other line, I nearly fainted. She had some births coming up and needed some assistance. I had become a certified doula (birth assistant) and this was my in. We attended a couple of births together and then she told me her partner was leaving to start her own practice and she needed to recreate her own. She asked if I would be interested in joining her practice as an acupuncturist and doula. The universe had heard my plea. (Thank you Universe.) The position was not as her employee, but to run my own business under her clinic's name, together with another naturopath who was just starting out. Now I had guidance and companions on my path. So much was already there for me: the website, the business cards, the name.

Dr. L bought a new space and for a month we worked hard on creating atmosphere. We turned a former alarm-system office, built and obviously decorated in the 1970s, into a tropical cabana-style health center. I ordered needles and herbs and prepared for reopening day. We invited the whole building, thirty-six floors, and everyone we knew for a reception. And then it was there, opening day: I had one patient scheduled.

The first year paralleled the last two. It was sink or swim. I needed to get things up and running. Should I advertise in the yellow pages? No. Should I get a credit-card machine? Yes. Should I validate parking? Yes. General excise taxes? What the…? Between starting a business and stepping into the role of a professional acupuncturist, I felt like a guppy in the big blue sea. *Fake it till you make it*, became my morning mantra as I headed to the clinic. Confidence would come with experience but until then, I leaned on the motto.

I learned a lot from Dr. L during my time with her. She was one of the busiest practitioners I knew. She lived her work as a naturopathic doctor and midwife pretty much 24/7. She was incredibly busy, at times chaotic, but as soon as a patient walked through the door she was all smiles and it was genuine. She treated everyone like a sister or brother, and she said this was a conscious decision. It was different from the practitioner/patient boundaries I had learned about in practice management classes. There was no white coat. When patients walked in the door, they took off their shoes (this is Honolulu), grabbed a cup of tea and were home. She maintained a perfect balance of casualness, approachability and professionalism.

She was too busy to hold my hand but Dr. L was a source of inspiration and I was blessed to be in her presence. She once told me how much she made her first year and I was shocked at the figure. Her advice for a successful first year: saying "yes" to everything, every patient, every venue that needed a speaker, every class that needed a teacher, anything and everything that would further a career. So I jumped on board and did the same: "Yes, yes, yes."

My patient volume slowly grew, and by my second year, I had a side job supervising a NADA detox clinic at a drug rehab center, taught two introductory classes at a local acupuncture college, set up booths at different expos and events, and had given a few public talks (a huge feat for someone with a public-speaking phobia).

Towards the end of that second year, I got a call from an acupuncturist in town who was leaving for five months and needed someone to take over her patients while she was away. She had established herself as a fertility specialist. I would see her patients at her place or mine and get a fifty percent cut. Since she charged on the higher end, my share was not much less than what I charged at my own practice. Plus it doubled my patient volume. "Yes, yes, yes."

This is the period where I gained some confidence as a practitioner. I realized that although I lacked experience, I did have something to contribute: a simple bedside manner and an earnest desire to help restore balance and harmony. I had just spent two years under the most adored practitioner in the state and I had absorbed the ability to create a space that was, if not inviting, at least not threatening. It was a welcome change for many patients who were used to the sterility of the doctor's office.

When patients sit before me, I want them to feel I am a friend who can be of help on their journey. And as a friend, I listen and refrain from judging what they express vocally or physically. Whether it is the struggle to conceive a child, gain freedom from addiction or deal with the darkness of one's own mind, I am there only to witness and aid. Since I am not a Daoist master, I can only embrace a camaraderie with patients as we both strive to embody our higher selves.

I discovered that most fertility patients have been trying to conceive for a while before they resort to acupuncture. They have been through it all – hormone injections, intrauterine insemination, in vitro – in the hope of fulfilling one of life's primal functions. For a woman or man, the diagnosis of "infertile" is a tough blow to the ego and patients often arrive in despair. I try to alleviate the stress, put them on a path to balance and let them leave with something positive.

This is something that has become a major part of my practice. In school we are taught TCM diagnosis: liver blood deficiency, spleen qi deficiency, damp-phlegm in the lower burner. But who wants to hear they have damp-phlegm in their lower burner anyway? And what is a lower burner? Most practitioners can probably remember experiencing a health crisis during their first year of school when they began braving the treatments in the intern clinic. "What? I have lung and spleen qi deficiency? I knew I had problems but I didn't know it was this bad."

So I try my best to explain what I observe without using much Chinese medical terminology. I rely on more graspable words. "Your pulse feels like you're being spread a little thin," or, "It seems like your metabolism could use a little boost." I go beyond the definition of endometriosis and talk about stagnation, the need for the color green in our lives, the need to get up and move, and the need to let go of patterns that no longer serve us. And I try to leave them empowered.

At the end of my five months working with fertility patients, I had learned a lot and formed some strong bonds. And this led to my first professional conflict. When the acupuncturist returned, she wanted, as agreed upon, her patients back. I never foresaw this as a problem, but as it turned out, some of the patients did. Some had never even met her, had only had a phone consultation with her before being referred to me. Bonds had been formed, trust was established, and most patients were on very heavy doses of hormones. A patient called crying. It was two days before her IVF procedure, was I really not going to be there for her? I promised to be there. This act terminated my professional relationship with the returning acupuncturist.

It took a bit of soul searching but I finally arrived at a place of comfort with my decision. In fact, it inspired me to reexamine and define my own ethical standards. I did not want money or ego to be the center of my practice. I had always wanted a life that was directed toward helping and that would remain my goal. Ever since this experience, whenever I have had to take leave and refer patients, I never demand they return. I believe the world is plentiful and there is enough to go around, no matter how often I feel like my practice is struggling. Everyone should find the individual or technique that best fits them. I am good with patients that come to me and I am good with those that leave. We all have our paths to follow and I do my best to respect that.

This experience rerouted my vision of practice. One of the many alluring elements of Chinese medicine is its holistic framework. Mind, body and spirit are all connected, and I wanted to really acknowledge that. I feel that our culture separates religion and the spiritual parts of life from everyday living, and talking about it has acquired an almost taboo status. One of the reasons I started out in acupuncture, and had chosen a program rooted in Daoist principles, was that it fed my desire to understand and feel a spiritual connection. I know I am not alone in that need.

I have found most people who come for acupuncture are searching for something deeper than relief from physical pain, which is where Chinese medicine can be of so much value. I often tell patients that acupuncture is a subtle medicine, but the subtly is enormous. Small energetic shifts can lead to great life transformations. Most people want to feel balanced and whole, so being able to tap into energy through qi gong or acupuncture, suggest foods or prescribe herbs for specific conditions, or retrain someone to breathe correctly is an incredible gift.

Change is continual and my practice is no exception. In my third year, the NADA clinic lost its funding and closed. But as one door shuts others open: another NADA program emerged through a community clinic and I was offered a completely unrelated job on Saturdays at an integrated health clinic run by a doctor of internal medicine. It had two medical doctors, a couple of nurse practitioners, physical therapists, massage therapists, a psychotherapist, a chiropractor and an acupuncturist. It was another wonderful opportunity and different from my other experiences. I entered the world of insurance: no fault, workman's comp and the small population whose insurance plans cover acupuncture. The majority were victims of car accidents seeking pain relief. The rooms were booked, the clinic was busy.

It was a big change. My own practice, because it was affiliated with naturopaths and the birthing community, drew a clientèle that were already quite health conscious and willing to pay out of pocket. The medical clinic drew from a more mainstream population who most often were under an insurance plan. The clinic operated on a system that begins with an appointment with a doctor who diagnoses and prescribes a therapeutic protocol; usually a combination of acupuncture, physical therapy and massage two or three times a week for several weeks. The vast majority of issues are musculoskeletal and at times the job feels a bit like a factory line.

But in the first few weeks, I realized it created the perfect opportunity to practice being present. If I did not focus, I could easily turn into a factory technician just throwing needles in. I wanted to avoid that trap, so I rearranged my attitude. I remembered to be thankful – for the consistent patient load and needling experience the job provided. I also found that being a part of this kind of clinic exposed me to a population I probably would not otherwise have contact with. I was treating Samoans, Tongans, Chinese (Yes, a white girl treating Chinese. Who would have thought?), Hawai'ians and Koreans. The exposure was vast and I enjoyed the exchange. Finally, I found the setting of a clinic that integrates Eastern and Western medicine very interesting. There are disadvantages and benefits when attempting to integrate, but mostly it is a great dialogue and a fantastic avenue for more exposure for our field.

In my fourth year of practice, I finally had to learn the word "no." I was spread too thin. I had my own business, taught three classes at the acupuncture college, worked Saturdays at the integrated office, and, oh yeah, there was my family. Things kept stacking up: GE taxes in January, learning to correctly pronounce the acupuncture points in Chinese before I taught the first-year students, ordering herbs, and preparing for my talk on postpartum care at the natural baby store.

Around this time, I was offered a full-time job at the doctor's office. I accepted and felt relief and gratitude for the stability, but sentimental and apprehensive about letting go of my own practice.

As I reflect back, I can see successes and failures along the way. In one sense, I am proud to have gained so much experience in my first few years out of school. In another, I can see how my divided attention hindered my ability to get my business up and running to a sustainable level. With more time, I would have devoted it to organizing, producing more pamphlets, attending more networking events, giving more lectures, meeting more doctors, revamping our website, sending out patient birthday cards, and on and on. But the reality is I did not have this time. I have many personal responsibilities outside work that need equal if not more attention. So for now, I will listen to the healer within who is saying, "Your pulse feels like you're spread too thin," and aim to re-balance. And when my personal load lightens, I look forward to once again recreating my own practice.

So for all the new and emerging practitioners out there, I wish you luck and blessings on this wonderful, wonderful journey.

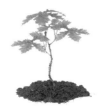

PART OF THE COMMUNITY
BY DAVID LESSEPS

I started TCM school three weeks after my son was born. For the first nine months I worked thirty hours a week at a grocery store, went to school full-time and changed diapers at night. The pace eased up a bit over time as larger student loans allowed me to spend more time with family and studying. Earning my masters degree took four years and approximately $90,000 in student loans. At the end of those four years I was unemployed, in debt and not entirely sure if my family could continue to pay rent for our one-bedroom apartment in San Francisco. Fortunately, I had stumbled upon a plan.

In my last year of school I heard about a new phenomenon called community acupuncture (CA). This approach to running an acupuncture clinic treats patients in large open rooms, four or more patients per hour, with sliding scale fees determined by the patient. I remember seeing a photograph of a room full of patients sitting in reclining La-Z-Boy chairs and wondering just exactly what was going on. After a little research I realized I had discovered something beautiful – an acupuncture clinic that I could afford to go to as a patient. Unfortunately, a CA clinic did not yet exist in San Francisco. But I now had a plan of what I was going to do with my acupuncture license. Six months after getting licensed and with two partners, Circle Community Acupuncture opened in September 2008.

Circle CA is located in San Francisco's South of Market neighborhood. We are nestled in a mixed residential and industrial district populated with bars, nightclubs, homes, cafes, printing presses, auto mechanics, welders, bail bondsmen, restaurants and a strip mall. The clinic is in a 1,200-square-foot storefront on a busy street close to a highway exit ramp. We are open seven days a week from 10 a.m. to 7 p.m. weekdays and noon to 5 p.m. on weekends. A total of five acupuncturists, one paid office manager and a small army of work-trade front desk helpers staff the clinic.

The reception area is separated from the treatment room by a large bookshelf and folding screens. The front desk is an old wooden table I found on the street while still a student. Reception is furnished in a hodgepodge mix of Ikea chairs, a vintage coffee table, carpet tiles, plants, children's toys, and a selection of books and magazines. On the front door and around the reception area are multiple signs reminding patients to use whispers when communicating.

On the other side of our book collection is the heart of the clinic – the treatment room. It comprises eleven reclining chairs arranged in a circle around a central table piled with blankets and sheets. In the southwest corner of the room is a massage table and a small workstation with glass vacuum cups and various liniments. Along the back wall is the entrance to the restroom and a small storage closet. The treatment area is arranged to balance clinical functionality with patient comfort. The reclining chairs are covered in brightly patterned vintage sheets, and there are multiple workstations with needles, cotton balls, alcohol dispensers, hand sanitizer and medical sharps containers. Paintings from a local artist hang on the walls and one wall is painted neon green. Small globe-shaped accent lamps, fans and white noise generators are scattered around the room.

A Day in the Clinic

My day starts with preparing for the day's patients. I tidy up, vacuum, warm up water for tea, stock supplies and pull patient charts. It is the only time when the clinic is empty other than myself, and I enjoy the quiet. I usually take a few minutes to sit in one of the recliners in the treatment room and just soak it in. I picture the room as it will soon be – full of patients. I look over charts, think about what is ahead of me for the day and try to find some quiet inside myself. Finally, I put on music, plug in the white-noise machines, flip the open sign and unlock the door.

The first two patients are outside waiting. One is a weekly regular and the other has been to the clinic a few times but this will be my first time treating her. I greet them, let them know they can settle into the treatment chairs and head back to wash my hands. After getting my needles ready, I sit on a stool next to my first patient and check in with him.

He has been coming regularly once or twice a week for a few months now. He originally started coming for debilitating migraines, and as those have cleared up he uses acupuncture for health maintenance and preventing complications from the medication he is taking for HIV and hepatitis C. Recently, we have been focusing on neuropathy in his feet, and for the first time in ten years he has had some sensation in this area. We briefly chat about how he is doing and if he has any other complaints. He reports that his left foot has been aching but otherwise is doing well. I feel his pulse, confirm that he has eaten breakfast and insert his needles.

Treating him reminds me of how my relationship to patients has changed. Fresh out of school, I would have focused on one thing: his diseases. HIV and hep-C would have flashed and blinked like beacons on his health history form. I would have hit him with a barrage of questions about his blood work, medications, side effects, diet, sexual activity, etc. In my head he would have become a "complicated patient" as a result of his health history. In school and in talking to colleagues I had developed the idea that people with chronic diseases and multiple complaints are somehow more complicated than others. However, treating thousands of patients has slowly chipped away at this idea. I have learned that the way to treat patients is to simply listen to what ails them at the time and then give the best treatment you can offer.

Once during my student internship, a patient came into the clinic with a sore throat and cough. The patient was transgender and identified as male. My clinic supervisor insisted I ask him multiple questions about his menstrual cycle and any hormonal supplements he was taking. During this questioning process, he became clearly confused by the focus on his sex. It was a humiliating experience for both of us. In the eyes of the supervisor, the patient was wearing a label, which obscured the main reason he was there – to seek relief.

Slowly, I am learning to let go of seeing labels on my patients. It is hard to let go of the idea that someone has fibromyalgia, rheumatoid arthritis or ovarian cysts. But when I can just sit down and listen to what patients are experiencing, it is much easier to treat them. When today's patient first came to the clinic, I had reached the point where I could hear that he had a left-sided migraine affecting the shaoyang and yangming channels, instead of seeing a complicated case of HIV and hep-C.

I move on to the next patient. She is new to me. According to her chart, she has not been in for a few months and was previously treated for sciatica. When I check in with her, she reports the sciatica has not returned and she is seeking treatment for work-related stress and anxiety. I ask a few questions about the nature of the anxiety, her sleep and check her pulse. While I am getting needles ready, she also mentions she woke up with a slight headache this morning. I make a quick mental adjustment to my point selection and proceed to put in the needles. Since this is my first time working with her and she seems a little nervous, I keep the treatment simple, only four body points and two on the ears.

By this time, two more patients have arrived. One is a returning patient and the other is here for the first time. While the regular settles in, I greet the new patient and ask him to complete some paperwork. The door opens and in walks another regular. We wave hello to each other and she proceeds into the treatment room.

I return to the treatment room for the third patient of the day, who is now settled into a recliner. She says her throat has been sore for two days, and she has a cough and body aches. I feel her pulse, check her tongue and ask her to swallow and tell me how much her throat is bothering her. She reports that it is very scratchy and feels swollen. The treatment starts with bleeding LI1 followed by needling. I tell her I will have some herbal pills ready for her, make sure she is covered with blankets and leave her to rest.

The next patient is a friend from outside the clinic who recently had surgery for endometriosis. She has not ovulated since and is still experiencing some pain. We quickly discuss her treatment goals and her most recent visit to a gynecologist. I ask her to come in twice a week until her cycle starts again and we talk about how long this might take. Then it is tongue, pulse and needles.

I quickly scan the room to make sure everyone is still resting before heading to the reception area to check on my new patient. By this time Bridget, the front-desk receptionist for the day, has arrived and is getting the new patient's paperwork into a chart. I quickly look it over, greet him and take him into the consultation room.

This "room" is actually a small corner of the reception area screened off by curtains. It is crowded with two chairs, three file cabinets, the day's charts, paperwork, a floor lamp and my lunch. Hanging on the walls are our diplomas, licenses, a painting that a patient made for the clinic, and some of my son's dragon drawings. While we take our seats, I give him a quick orientation to the clinic. We discuss the need for whispering, how to check in during return visits, where the bathroom is, and other bits and pieces before moving on to his reasons for coming in. Our intake sheets have room for patients to list three main complaints. His intake form shows he is experiencing knee and foot pain from a running injury, and that he has a long history of depression. I ask him about the running injury, such as when and where he feels pain. We talk about his depression and what he has done to treat it. He says he is not taking any medication, but meets with a student therapist once a week. After a few questions about some digestive complaints and his sleep, we discuss how often he should come and what progress to expect over time. Then we head to the treatment room.

This whole interaction takes about five minutes. When I was in school, we spent thirty minutes or longer on new patient intakes. It took me a while to let go of the herbal-based *zang-fu* diagnostic approach I was taught in school, which required in-depth questioning across several physiological systems. The habit of the long intake has required a lot of conscious effort to shake off. In the beginning, I found myself habitually asking patients about diet and bowel movements when their chief complaint was low back pain. Knee pain was not just knee pain, it was kidney deficiency; depression was liver qi stagnation or heart-kidney disharmony. Having now studied meridian-based acupuncture systems, I quickly know how to treat knee pain just by knowing where it hurts. With depression, I want to know if they are sleeping and eating, how much energy they have, and what their pulse feels like. Also, as I have gained confidence in the benefits of acupuncture, I have learned to let go of the long-winded intakes. It has taken a while to get to this point; not because I have become a great practitioner who can discern the heart of a patient at a glance, but because I have learned to trust the simple fact that acupuncture helps people to feel better. I have had to learn that acupuncture is beneficial to patients regardless of whether I have deduced the perfect diagnosis. Something wonderful and almost magical happens to a person when they receive acupuncture and the body is allowed to heal itself. I learned to trust in this by watching it in action day after day.

Back in the treatment room, one of the patients is awake and her eye contact lets me know she is ready to leave. I pull her needles and remind her to come back in a few days. Another patient catches my attention and asks for a second blanket, which I cover her with before starting with the new patient's treatment. After his needles are in place I return to the consultation room to do some charting while the most recent patients settle into their recliners.

The treatment room is now full of sleeping people. It has lost the quiet feeling of pre-opening and is now filled with the sounds of sleep, white noise machines, ambient music, footsteps, the occasional cough or sniffle, and Bridget taking care of phone calls and paperwork. All voices are whispers and none of the noises are loud or abrupt, but the room practically hums with human presence. There is something magical about a room full of resting adults receiving acupuncture, and the times when I remember to stop and take it in are some of the happiest of my workday.

Of course it was not like this when Circle CA first opened. On our first day we had three patients. I remember the first time I saw fifteen patients in a shift: I finished the day completely wiped out and frazzled by the experience. I had struggled to keep on schedule and felt like I was running in circles. It has taken time and experimentation to allow the clinic to grow to its current level of activity. I have had to learn both how to be a practitioner and how to be a business owner.

School left us with a shamefully non-existent education for running a business. My partners and I have had to learn how to negotiate a lease, and write a business plan and partnership agreement, as well as figure out bookkeeping and marketing strategies. We have been through a partnership change, tax troubles and employees leaving. The biggest lesson has been to wear both hats – clinician and business owner – but to not let them interfere with one another. When I am at the clinic, it is my job to worry about whether we are busy enough, but I cannot let anxiety seep into my interactions with patients. During a clinic shift, my focus must be on listening to and treating patients, and facilitating a smooth flow of activity. When making business decisions, I have to make sure that they will keep the clinic running smoothly and self-sustaining. If the clinic does not run well, we will not have patients; and without patients, I am not an acupuncturist.

My shift continues and by the end I have seen twenty-one patients in five hours. I finish by filling out charts and waiting for resting patients to finish. I greet my clinic partner and another acupuncturist as they arrive and start treating the evening patients. I straighten up the consultation room, clean my needle station, wash my hands, say good-bye to Bridget and take off. Tomorrow morning I start it all again.

Being a Community Acupuncturist

When I was an intern in my last year of school, if I was lucky I would see four patients in a shift of about four hours. Much of that time was spent doing extensive patient interviews, tracking down clinic supervisors, putting together herbal packages in the pharmacy and filling out paperwork. Very little of it was actually spent needling people. In the first three months at Circle CA, I treated more patients than I did in my entire four years of school. On a busy day, I schedule six return patients an hour and if I get walk-ins that can become seven or eight. This does not leave a lot of time for unnecessary actions.

I have had to learn to keep my intakes and diagnoses focused. Most of my post-school acupuncture education has been focused on learning the meridian-based acupuncture styles of Richard Tan and Master Tung. These styles focus on identifying which meridians are sick and using this information to determine point selection. Before I even say hello to a patient, I have begun my assessment of their condition. I am looking at their posture, skin tone, eye contact, and general level of awareness and activity. When I sit down next to them and whisper a greeting, I start to feel their pulse. I am checking quickly to determine if they are excess or deficient, rapid or slow, tight or soft. I ask them how they are feeling, what they are currently experiencing and what changes, if any, they have noticed since the previous treatment. Usually, before we are finished talking, I have decided which points I am going to use.

Many of the patients at our clinic come two or more times a week. During intakes I am also learning little snippets of their life. I learn about their jobs, loves, families, anxieties, drugs of choice, cravings and desires. We tell each other about special dinners or events from the day before. This information adds up and over time we develop a relationship that is more than a list of ailments and complaints. We know each other's moods and personalities. This may not directly help me in diagnosing a complaint, but it has taught me much about the human condition.

I see an incredible spectrum of people at the clinic. Our patients are bakers, baristas, waiters, grocery stockers, attorneys, students, sex workers, pot farmers, therapists, social workers, electricians, unemployed, artists, nurses, teachers, bus drivers, labor organizers, local politicians and pretty much any other career you can think of. On any given day, I will see patients who identify as heterosexual, homosexual, transgender, male or female. In walk African Americans, Asian Americans, European Americans, Latin Americans and recent immigrants. Patients speak English, Spanish, Cantonese, Mandarin, Tagalog, Portuguese, Italian and languages I can only guess at. They walk in covered in sweat from riding their bikes while others cruise in on wheelchairs or using canes. Some patients can fill out their health history in two minutes, others need it read to them because of visual impairments. Because of the varied mix of cultural, ethnic, gender and class perspectives that come to our clinic everyday, I cannot rely on verbal communication alone. Many times an intake comprises of feeling a pulse, eye contact, a smile and a hand on the shoulder.

As a community acupuncturist, I have learned that it is my job to understand the word "community." When I walk around the city on my day off, I often run into patients: We wave to each other, give each other a smile or stop and chat. I often see people whose name I cannot remember, but I remember the month they came in for help with severe morning sickness.

When patients come to the clinic, each one has something that is bothering them. For some it is as simple as a hangover from a night of drinking while others might suffer from debilitating migraines or frequent panic attacks. When they sit in the chair and talk to me, they can tell me as much or as little about their condition as they like. I listen to them and experience it with them for a moment. Once the needles are in place and they enter a nice acu-nap, they are sharing that time with everyone else in the room. In my eyes, this is community.

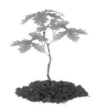

WARFARE IN SPRINGTIME
BY JOHN RENNA

October 8, 2004:

My first patient of the week was a woman in her mid-40s. She has chronic insomnia and has recently experienced panic attacks with anxiety. She cannot mow the lawn or play with her daughter without her heart racing. She literally has not slept soundly in the past nine months while her husband has been deployed in Iraq.

My second patient was in her 30s and was rear-ended in an accident and cannot work for several weeks. She has severe headaches, as well as neck and back pains. Her husband is also deployed to Iraq. She has no one to help take care of her daughter while she is incapacitated with injuries. She said she speaks with her husband briefly on the phone every other day. He has not been allowed to say much due to restrictions after the Abu Ghraib prison scandal. All cameras have been confiscated, and telephone calls and emails are monitored. According to her, all he can say is, "I am ashamed of being a soldier," and that atrocities are still being committed every day.

My fifth patient was the wife of a soldier. She had not slept in the week since she learned her husband was killed in Iraq.

This was just one week....

*   *   *

I do not write this as an antiwar piece. If anything, closer to the opposite. But because my early years in practice coincided with the war in Iraq, and my office sat barely fifteen minutes from one of the largest army bases in the nation, the war cannot help but be part of my story.

Mental anguish such as these three patients experienced solidified to me the TCM notion regarding health and the seven emotions. "Solidified" is not even the right word – it screamed it. Several patients seemed to have all seven rolled into a tight ball in their gut. "What is my diagnosis?" they would ask. Inside I was thinking, "Well, you have a complicated case we call stagnation of joyangerfearfrightpensiveness-melancholy." Or I would bite my tongue to keep from saying something like, "You are choking on a bitter pill called war." But no one in the armed forces – neither soldier nor spouse – would accept that comment, since fighting is what they had been preparing for, and people told me that repeatedly. Because I never knew my military families before the battles began, I had to try to discern how much existed prior to all the upheaval. That meant asking the right questions – one of the most fundamental points to practice.

But before I get into that, I should explain where these patients came from. Yes, my clinic was just a short drive from an army base – and a lovely drive as well, through the low mountains of Hawai'i as they rolled into the sea. But I also saw numerous naval officers, air force members and even marines from a base nearly two hours away. They popped in the door in full military dress, said hello, then ducked into the restroom to change into "civvies." They were simply willing to come, which is no small feat considering one of the few big perks of being in the military is fully covered health care, and I charged cash. So where did these patients come from? Mainly from one abundant, generous source I affectionately called The Mouth. She was not my only master referrer, but one of the greatest. Most practitioners have likely had at least one, and I was blessed with four in my first year or so of professional practice.

Mouths are those endearing patients who do not just refer a patient or two, but refer many, and many good ones. They do not just write down your office number on a napkin, but clean you out of business cards and hand them out personally. They tell you about people they refer, giving you an idea of what to expect, or leave a brief email or phone message asking, "Can you book me for two treatments, because I am bringing so-and-so along." But the message is not really a request, it is more a statement: the "can you" is a polite formality. In short, we should be paying these Mouths instead of vice versa!

This particular referral machine was the wife of an officer. She basically had three jobs on base: welcoming newly arrived families – mostly those under her husband's extensive command – comforting families of fallen or injured soldiers, and working to maintain sanity on base by teaching yoga and fitness. She was often the first shoulder to cry on, and came to me for recharging. Secured by the confidentiality of my office, she could unload her own grief, her own stress, even sometimes letting slip military tidbits not meant for my ears, and all of what she said revealed the humanity and compassion involved in times of war. I massaged tension from her shoulders, vented points with needles, prescribed herbs for strength and sanity, and, perhaps most importantly, listened. To me, the act of listening should overshadow the ten questions. And I was told repeatedly over the years that what separated me from many other doctors and practitioners was my ability to listen.

This is interesting to reflect on, because in school I distinctly remember teachers, especially the biomedical instructors, stressing the different aspects of questioning. In my first few semesters, we had classes entirely devoted to learning how to use time efficiently and effectively through precision questioning – a case unraveled and a diagnosis made with just three questions, the scalpel always paring things down further and further. Asking, pointing, prodding, directing... In clinic our intake forms were crammed with dozens of questions, most of which I eventually removed from my own forms. I cannot recall a single class where we were taught how to listen. Time, we were told, is your enemy.

But listening takes time. Perhaps the early years of practice are supposed to be slow, with fewer patients, so we have the chance to listen, to nurture this skill. Mistakes happen in haste far more often than great successes.

When I sold my practice after seven years, I was seeing as many as fourteen patients a day solo, without office staff. Because my listening skills had been honed, time was not my enemy, and I could navigate the sea of information deftly. Because I listened, I needed to ask less – and paying attention was the key to discerning what to ask. I used the time I could have spent talking to let my patients say what they felt they needed to. This made a profound difference in shaping my practice and it influenced the people drawn to me.

Although I feel that engaging with patients always drains qi, speaking burns it quicker than listening. Sure, often my inexperienced mind was busy inside thinking about the next step, maybe confused about a particular symptom, or trying to remember something heard or read years before. But as in the Buddhist Eightfold Path, right understanding and right thoughts come before right speech. So I listened, and that reputation grew.

Nearly all of my military patients had qi constraint caused by emotional issues, which then exacerbated their physical complaints. Initially, I did not approach the medicine from this direction. In fact, I doubt I could name all seven classical emotions when I graduated. I knew it intellectually, but did not deeply understand it, or even care to. I originally practiced a straightforward, hands-on TCM: lots of herbs and lots of needles with shiatsu and physio-type therapy worked in. But as I practiced, I watched fixed pains unwind virtually unaided as emotions were released on my table. Even if few words were spoken, there was no hiding tear stains on the pillowcase. Anguish sinks strength, anxiety exhausts it, as does sleeplessness. A lack of power slows movement and leads to stagnation. Fear grips muscles and squeezes tears from the body. Tears are one of the strongest examples of this connection between soma and neuma, body and spirit: something physical manifesting from the emotional. No classroom or intern clinic could show this like having the time to really listen and observe, where the energy is just between myself and the patient.

So almost every time someone presented with physical pain, I learned to listen closely for ways to release constraint through the mind, not just with needles and hands. Laughter, asking about children – any small thing to bring light and joy to the moment. Since Hawai'i is such a transient place, where so many people are from somewhere else, I often said, "Tell me the three best things about living in Hawai'i, in no particular order." A question like this directs a person to the realm of hope, perhaps triggering memories that transcend present suffering.

Sometimes, perhaps often, the diagnosis is not really clear until the treatment is a success, "hindsight is 20/20" as the saying goes. It is not exactly accidental, because we likely have followed a certain path, but the picture is not clear until one looks back. Looking back on the physical pains hanging on these military establishment patients, three-quarters dissolved completely once a loved one came home or was heard from after weeks incommunicado. Did they really have pain, or did they simply need caring for in the interim?

On base, SSRI and NSRI drugs – Paxil, Effexor, Zoloft and Prozac – were handed out like candy, often in combination with sleeping pills or pain meds. I also frequently saw Lexapro, Celexa, Seroquel and Abilify. Yet counseling services, though technically available, were far too understaffed to meet the immense and sudden needs of hundreds of wives, girlfriends, a few men and loads of children, whose loved ones had just deployed to or returned from a war zone. So just by listening, my reputation grew.

But an available ear and holistic counseling were not the only things that helped my popularity with this group. Another was herbs. Still another is so difficult to talk about I hesitate to even mention it. So the easy one first: herbology.

I love herbs! I began studying herbal medicine six years before starting acupuncture school. Needles are brilliant, simple, effective: I greatly respect them. But I truly love herbs more. In practice, the income from them can create a solid base of earning – at least in the United States and Asia where they are less rigorously regulated than in much of Europe. And I was the only practitioner in my community who practiced them proficiently. Neighboring acupuncturists actually sent their patients to me for herbal consults and products. In fact, on more than one occasion I treated a fellow acupuncturist while a patient referred by that practitioner was in my waiting room. It created some interesting triangular relationships, but never in a negative way. On the contrary, I had healthy working relationships with all my competition, and urge all budding practitioners to have as much interaction with their peers as possible. Having had training in herbs, I would never run a practice on needles and bodywork alone.

How this relates to my military families goes back to those antidepressants and anti-anxiety medications I mentioned above. No patient liked them. Even if effective, just the idea of being on medication was often very distasteful, exacerbating feelings of helplessness and depression. Drugs could also dull responses toward loved ones at a time when richer emotional connections were what was actually needed. And the prescribing doctor was routinely quite vague about how long a patient would be on the medication. Some experienced intense side effects: tremors, sweating, headaches, fatigue and flat affect. I may be preaching to the choir when I say this class of drugs has gaping shortcomings, but because they were so ubiquitous, I was forced to get to know them extremely well.

My TCM education included pharmacology classes taught by two nurses. Adequate training, but it by no means made me proficient. That level of knowledge works for most practitioners, as most in the West start TCM training partially out of rebellion toward Western allopathic medicine, and often specifically against pharmaceuticals. I know I did, though today much of my angst has evolved with experience, and hope does shine through because I can more easily recognize and give credit to the good doctors and researchers working hard to make a difference.

But one day a patient challenged me to find an herbal replacement for her medication – Zoloft. She hated it! And it was the third medication her physician had tried her on. That afternoon, this patient said something to me I have repeated to a hundred patients since, it was such a gift. She said, "As long as I'm basically this doctor's guinea pig, trying a new drug every few weeks to see what happens, I might as well trade this process for herbs, which are safer."

I could have cried I was so pleased. We spend so much time and effort trying to get this point across to the public, so when someone says it back to you, you want to shout with joy. I might have actually shed a tear when she followed this by saying, "And I trust you – you actually listen." It was at that point I knew I had crossed a threshold, achieved something I had worked long and hard for.

Faced with her challenge, I began an undertaking that forever changed my practice: I learned to acquire, read and understand pharmacological data – at first just for this class of drugs but eventually for nearly any medication a patient came in on. Medscape is an excellent online resource regarding drugs and interactions. With a patient resting comfortably on a table I could hit the computer and quickly fill in any knowledge gaps about their meds, or catch updates on current drug news. I also enhanced my endocrinology knowledge and delved deeper into understanding herbal combinations; both in classical and modern terms by actively seeking out herbs' chemical components while also referring to my favorite nineteenth-century translation of the ancient Chinese herbal classic, Shen Nong Ben Cao. I took online continuing education courses for medical doctors, even though I received no actual credit for it. This gave me linguistic power when speaking with both patients and their physicians, but perhaps more importantly, it allowed me to see things from the point of view of the allopathic doctor.

Biomedical journals, so unlike TCM publications, are littered with stories of failure and humility. But each failure is seen as a valuable learning experience and a step toward improvement. The two fields do have drastically different views of valid research, but even with that in mind, our profession does itself a disservice by glittering the pages of its publications almost exclusively with positive anecdotes and glowing results, when we all know failures are common.

From this point forward, prescription meds never scared, confused, repelled or intimidated me. I was able to identify and discuss my patients' medications with them, observe side effects more clearly, and know with confidence when to send them back to their prescribing doctor for possible changes. Others may not want to do this, but I rarely hesitated to prescribe herbs on top of drugs – because I understood them. And lastly, I accepted every patient's challenge to wean them off prescription medication in exchange for herbs, and then with luck, eventually off of any daily regimen be it holistic or allopathic.

Returning to this patient and her Zoloft, I had heard a rumor that this drug was synthesized in part from a key component of the herb *shi chang pu*. I have never been able to verify this rumor, unfortunately, but that does not really matter. This plant, and at least two similar ones, have historically been used for lifting people's moods. Blended appropriately, it helped form a fantastic base for a line of three formulas I developed with the help of my patients: one for depression, another for anxiety and the last for combination disorders causing qi exhaustion, such as from sleep loss. The formulas were a hit. I was able to get most of my military patients off their depression and related drugs, while helping them through months or years of crisis revolving around a vicious and confusing war.

One of my favorite bumper stickers reads, "It will be a great day when schools have all the money they need and the military has to hold a bake sale to buy a bomber." I was not born a pacifist but I became one as a teen – in a shout in the street kind of way. This gratefully gave way to a more meditative stance, but the underlying belief remained the same: I refused to support any organization that trained human beings to kill other human beings. It was a line I used at eighteen years old when military recruiters first began calling my home and I never changed it. I have insulted service members with it and nearly been pummeled physically because of it.

When I began my practice in a community that was world famous for its surfing, I tried to convince other practitioners in the building to work together to market our services to the water-sports crowd. Our center had a variety of separate businesses in various healing disciplines from rolfing to yoga, Hawai'ian healing, massage and personal fitness. Upon hearing my ideas, the other practitioners groaned and rolled their eyes. I was newer to the area than my colleagues. "Been there, done that," was their tone. Late for appointments, show up liquored or stoned, forget their wallets, underemployed, don't follow directions... and then turn right around to repeat whatever action got them injured in the first place. This was not a pool of patients worth actively seeking out. But I pushed ahead and did it anyway on my own, much to my misfortune.

A few wished to direct things towards the nearby army base, but nothing got off the ground, in part because a few of us stuck our noses up in regards to the war and thus to those involved in it. Most military folk are proud and want to go fight; something I could not fathom and a type of energy I did not want to surround myself with. We were also faced with the daunting, grinding gears of the bloated military system: questions unanswered, calls not returned or endlessly redirected.

But my first Mouth – and the many patients that stemmed from her – taught me lessons beyond anything school had offered, and effectively shattered my metallic rigidity. A healer is supposed to have empathy and compassion, so how could one possibly hold these notions back from any particular group or selfishly direct them to a hand-picked few? Not only that, but my beliefs and arrogance had shut me out of a huge contingency of nearby business potential. When a soldier, officer, or their relation did come, I had a choice. I could neglect follow-up, abbreviate treatments, offer slimmer service, be cold and impersonal – or I could treat them with empathy, like any other person.

When I gave in and acted with all the compassion I could muster, my practice blossomed, it flowed like running water and never stopped. I quit taking new patients for the first time on my two-year anniversary because business had grown beyond my strength. When I let go and let nature decide the course, I met some amazing and rewarding people – not patients, but people – each unique and deserving as much as the rest. Until the day I sold my practice after seven years, the military continued to fuel between fifty to sixty percent of my practice, and dozens were faithful patients for years.

But there is one more subject I encountered in my first years of practice I would like to talk about: the most personal and painful one.

*   *   *

It is not yet seven o'clock when my phone rings. This is a.m., not p.m., and I am still in bed. Too early for phone conversations so I let it go to voice mail. Fifteen minutes later while shaving, it rings again. Figuring it must be important, I answer. On the other end of the line is a familiar voice, but not in a familiar tone: "What's this I hear about

Lyn leaving her husband for you!" she shouts. My reply is stunted, stunned, "Um... uh, what?!" On the other end of the line was The Mouth, who had referred Lyn to me.

"I got off the phone with Lyn a few minutes ago and she says she is leaving Michael for you, that you are okay with this, that you two were meant to be together!" comes the frantic, angry response.

*   *   *

Transference, it is called in the Diagnostic and Statistical Manual of Mental Disorders when a patient or client becomes attracted to the caregiver. They become attached to the attention, listening and possibly touch; grow fond of the safe, secure, nurturing environment. These things are likely missing from their lives, or the caregiver is linked in their minds to a caring person from long ago. People like this interpret professional encounters as though they were personal.

I should have seen it coming with Lyn (not her or her husband's real names) – and with the two other married patients who professed attraction to me. Perhaps I did see it but belittled the scale or significance. Or profoundly worse, maybe I liked the flattery; or the income, as these patients were faithful regulars.

How did this happen? I had taken a course in my final year of TCM college called "Psychology for Patient Counseling." One of my first biomedical instructors was a young pediatric psychiatrist who constantly rerouted his classes to subjects about psychological issues. And fifteen years prior, I helped found one of the country's first peer-counseling centers in a high school. I have always kept current with the psychological sciences, so basically there was no excuse for me to have missed these brewing problems.

But transference, I was to learn, is particularly prevalent in the military among women whose significant others are stationed overseas for months at a time. Often in the armed forces, couples commit far too young and far too soon, rushed by a pending move or transfer far away. Korea, Guam, Philippines, from California to South Carolina... Iraq. I had a male patient who married a woman he had dated for just four weeks because she was soon headed to Iraq. He was retired army and his first wife left him the month he returned from his own tour in the Middle East.

Until finally leveling off in 2009, during the Afghan and Iraq wars U.S. military divorce rates were the highest they had been in the history of the armed forces, according to Department of Defense statistics.

One patient told me a third of his platoon ended their marriages while in Iraq. These "domestic casualties" are one of the less discussed aspects of war: divorce, infidelity and schools overwhelmed by emotionally burdened children from these broken homes. Not only were separation rates skyrocketing, according to my sources, scores of women left behind were having affairs while their husbands overseas were also having affairs. Unfortunately, these issues were loud and clear in the military patients I saw, including their children.

So I should have seen it coming. There are standard and legal practices when transference occurs. Needless to say, after Lyn I got on the ball quickly! But it still happened: Thank you cards became more personal, emails edged closer to that line, gifts were more extravagant, disrobing became too easy, or I was asked to treat or check near genital areas when it was not necessary. (I should clarify that in Hawai'i it is common for patients to bring doctors and dentists small gifts – food, gift cards, small things for the office.)

Was it me then? I wrote earlier that I initially had a very hands-on practice. I began herbs years before starting TCM, but even before that I had trained in shiatsu. I like to palpate points, let my hands work more than my mouth, and move joints and fascia around. For a woman whose husband is overseas for almost a year, returns for nine months, then is gone for another year, it is obvious that being touched by a man can be enjoyable – even if it is being misinterpreted. And then there is the caring factor, the personal nature of medical questions, especially our holistic questioning that ranges from matters involving family and friends to menstruation and sleep. I could dedicate as much as thirty minutes to listening, while inexperienced or overwhelmed military doctors barely had five minutes. Our local army hospital was staffed largely with doctors fresh out of internship who had joined the military to get their school loans forgiven.

I decided something more had to change.

I began with adjustments in body language. I stood more or sat farther away with more time behind the desk. I took pulses while standing – never sitting in front of a patient or on the table next to them, which seemed too casual. Like most practitioners, I loathe charting, but my notes gained accuracy and comprehension. For one it gave my presence a more professional air, but detailed notes also offered potential legal protection if any questions arose. "Yes, I touched her buttocks, but because the patient complained of sciatic pain." I hugged less, subtly mentioned my relationships more, such as something my girlfriend and I had done over the weekend, and after I got married I wore my wedding ring more, which unfortunately hindered some massage techniques. I also started practicing more distal styles of acupuncture. After all, it is well-established in the Chinese literature that male doctors had as little physical contact with female patients as possible. Some credit this restraint for the creation of radial pulse taking, and others say the five transport points gained their popularity through only being able to needle the hands, feet, wrists and ankles.

But one thing I did not do was stop seeing any patient who professed attraction to me or whom I suspected of it. To this day I do not know if that was a mistake. But I gave each woman a choice. The married ones I invited to the office at lunchtime, establishing a window of time but with a limit, as afternoon patients were scheduled. I made tea and then reinforced the professional nature of our relationship. I offered referrals to other acupuncturists or family counselors. I told them I had no problem continuing to see them professionally, but they would have to decide.

All continued. And they all gave the same reason, "Your treatments are helping, so I wish to continue." No matter the reason, I saw them again and again – one of them even up until the day I sold my practice years later. The three married women all remained with their husbands, two others went on to greatly improved family lives, and one at least did no worse by my estimation. And by continuing to see them, I think it perhaps helped them see what they were doing, helped clarify their lives and actions, see why the marriages were crumbling. I ran into "Lyn" a few years later and she said, "I don't know what I was thinking back then – to think I would've left my husband for you!" I smiled. I might have been insulted, but I could not have been more pleased.

I sold my Hawai'i practice in 2010 after seven years in the same office. I had completely outgrown my two treatment rooms and was just plain tired after four years of graduate school followed immediately by the seven of full-time practice. I had started from scratch: One day, one patient at a time, and simply persisted. I found regular office hours to be a big key to success – being there even with no patients scheduled – being there for walk-ins, last-minute needs, herb refills, etc.

With the practice sold, I took eight months off to travel with my wife across the United States, England, India, Thailand, and finally New Zealand where I now live and am growing a new practice. I truly love The Medicine, and as I have had teachers still practicing into their 70s, I may very well do the same. I also hope to embark on a doctorate in public health here, comparing treatment outcomes in the United States with its private system of health care to those in a country with a national system such as New Zealand. Since 2007, I have also traveled annually to Burma to teach and treat through the nonprofit organization Vipassana Hawai'i.

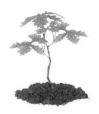

LEARNING THE BASICS
BY SUZANNE ROBIDOUX

After finishing a four-year masters degree program in the United States and managing my own clinic for a couple of years in Canada, I realized I had a deep desire to learn more about the ancient science and art of Chinese medicine. At the time, it seemed like the only place I could go was Asia, which meant my first step was the daunting task of learning Mandarin. But desire was stronger than fear of the unknown, so I dropped everything, quit my job and my relationship, sold my car, moved all my things into storage, found a job online, and moved to Taiwan.

I settled in the southern city of Tainan, where the Lonely Planet said there were more temples than 7-Elevens. I arrived, settled in at my new job, and within a week had found a tai ji quan and tuina massage teacher who two years later became my shifu. I started private Chinese lessons right away, which was a necessary and challenging reality for basic survival.

I studied Chinese medicine in clinics located in the city's alleys. The Taiwanese people and their traditional culture charmed me. For three years, I studied with skilled traditional teachers of qi gong, martial arts and Chinese medicine, some who combined all three in their practices. It was a special time and I learned some of the deeper aspects of Chinese medicine. By the end of three years, however, I felt it was time to head to the mainland and learn from the birthplace of our medicine. I chose the oldest acupuncture university and applied to their doctoral program. Amazingly, they accepted me and a month later I set out for Nanjing, against all of the warnings of my friends.

I arrived in the middle of August. If you ever go to Nanjing in summer, you will understand why it is called one of the "four ovens" of China. My plane landed at 2 a.m. and it was nearly hot enough to give me heatstroke. As I listened numbly to the taxi driver, I gazed out the window at men with their shirts rolled up to expose their round bellies, spitting in the street. This was a different world from the tropical island paradise I had just left. Still, I was determined to find a teacher who could show me the depths of Chinese medicine.

The next day I arrived at the university campus, hopeful and happy. But as I walked through the gray and broken-down buildings, I thought a bomb had just gone off and no one was left to pick up the pieces. I asked for directions to the building for foreign students, but no one would respond. So I continued walking deeper in, past barking dogs and corners that smelled of urine. Eventually, I found a shy but willing student who guided me to one of the buildings in the back. The place reeked of rats, but the student told me I needed to go to the sixth floor. So I walked into the dark elevator and was shocked when it actually worked.

Stepping out, I was in a completely different world. The lights worked. Windows were new. There were nice carpets, air-conditioned classrooms and cushioned chairs. This was the administration office and where short-term classes for foreigners were held. However, when they handed me my schedule, I saw that those of us in the full-time, three-year program studied with the Chinese students. This meant we would be in classrooms with broken windows, no air conditioning in the boiling hot summers and no heat of any kind in winter, when temperatures hit well below zero. I remember clutching hot water bottles during night classes in the winter so I would not freeze on my little wooden chair.

All the full-time foreign students were put together with a few Chinese students. We were mostly Koreans and Taiwanese, with one Japanese, one Cuban, one Mexican, one Brazilian and me. The first hour of every topic was the same message, "Chinese medicine is part of Chinese culture and isn't meant to be learned by foreigners." After hearing the first teacher say this, I felt shocked and angry, but later realized these were very traditional teachers, and eventually was able to keep listening without giving it a second thought. It was similar to the introduction I had received in martial arts. I saw it as a kind of test, to see if we had the determination to learn something outside the realm of our own cultures.

I continued with my lessons and held onto my hope of finding a doctor who had mastered the skills of Chinese medicine. But the first semester was so full of paperwork and administrative obligations I almost forgot why I had come. In the second half of the year, I was told I needed to find an adviser. I looked long and hard, and finally chose our school's previous headmaster, who came highly recommended by a good friend and had perfect credentials. She had spent time abroad teaching TCM in Myanmar and seemed perfect for me. How could I have known the difficulties that were to come?

Looking back on the three years of torture, I can see it was nothing personal, and perhaps even pretty standard for a teacher-student relationship in China. I do not want to sound like an ungrateful foreigner, but after being chronically lied to about deadlines and working standards, after being denied any help whatsoever in every and all situation, and after having my papers stolen by the same people who were supposed to have been helping me, I guess something snapped. Eventually I went outside the structure of the university to learn what I needed to, and adapted to the situation as best I could to become the practitioner I wanted to be.

Language and cultural issues were the least of my worries. The lack of connections is every foreign student's worst enemy. Nonetheless, I was not about to quit. Looking back now, I am grateful I persevered. Somehow through all the administrative confusion, the constant numbing noise of the city and the frequent bouts of food poisoning, I found a few very meaningful people who made it all worthwhile. Right in the middle of the chaos and distress, in the polluted air and live-or-die lifestyle, they were there, quietly and skillfully practicing the graceful art of Chinese medicine.

One of these amazing people was a kind and helpful doctor at a neurological hospital who I met during my internship. My adviser had solid connections and was in the middle of a research project on depression in the inpatient department. So I was fortunate and soon replaced a graduating student to become one of the practicing doctors in a clinical trial using acupuncture for severe depression with suicidal tendencies.

Every day we performed the same acupuncture protocol on these patients. Depression is taboo in China, so these people were often secretly administered to the hospital without their employers or families, sometimes even their spouses, ever knowing the real reason. We learned about the daily pressures they faced and their discontent. It was gratifying to gradually reduce their medication and then help them reintegrate with society under continued outpatient care. But after a few months, I found the treatment approach repetitive and limiting. I needed more stimulation.

One morning while leaving the hospital after my shift, I noticed a short female doctor in the outpatient acupuncture department. Dr. Lu was the only doctor in a room full of patients. If you have ever seen an acupuncture clinic in China, you know that patients come without appointments and line up until their turn comes. In this case, patients were lined up in the hallways and many had waited for hours.

I introduced myself to Dr. Lu and told her about the research project I was working on at the hospital. She knew of us, of course, and the program, but had no time for chitchat. I hung around and saw she was treating severe cases of hemiplegia, paralysis, Parkinson's and other neurological and spinal disorders mainly using scalp acupuncture. I offered to help, as it seemed she could use another set of hands. She did not even have time to accept before a patient's timer dinged, indicating it was time to remove the needles. She pointed to him and told me to remove the needles to make room for the next patient. And that is how my apprenticeship with Dr. Lu began.

From then on, I came to help Dr. Lu every morning at the hospital. Her schedule was packed with severe cases of post-stroke sequelae and other neurological diseases or emotional breakdowns. Dr. Lu had learned from a famous master of scalp acupuncture who used a variation of the Jiao cranial acupuncture technique. It was very effective. Patients received treatment every day, and most showed daily progress. There was also a clear evolution in the treatment protocol and slowly I got a handle on her techniques, but I still had a lot to learn.

About three months after I started training, a patient came in who had post-stroke aphonia. I had seen this treated many times since it was a fairly common symptom, but the protocol turned my stomach. It involved using a thick needle to violently prick the patient's tongue superficially until it bled profusely. Then you had to stretch out the patient's tongue and needle it more than one cun deep with a three-inch needle and stimulate it strongly while the patient cried in agony. It is possible I dreaded this procedure almost as much as the patients.

But on that day, Dr. Lu looked at me and handed me the three-inch needle. I took it, but could not bring myself to do it. When I hesitated, she got very angry. This usually friendly and joyful doctor became as hard and strict as a general. She told me, "If you want to be a good doctor, you need to be able to harden your heart when you have to. How can the xie qi (qi causing the disease) leave the patient if you show fear and hesitate?" She took the needle back and performed the treatment protocol with strength and confidence. This was very far from the painless treatments given in the United States, but sure enough, it proved effective and the patient was able to speak within three weeks.

I learned something that day that will stay with me forever. Until then, I had thought that being a good doctor meant not only being well-trained, but also being kind and compassionate. But that day I realized something important was missing. I also needed to strengthen my confidence in my technique so I could do what my patients needed without hesitation.

In Western societies, we usually associate Chinese medicine with alternative care or complementary medicine, which has an underlying soft, gentle, new-age feeling. But in China, it is a medicine, a science and an art. So, just like in Western medicine, one sometimes has to draw blood or do something that leaves a scar, such as with moxa, to bring a patient back to health. That day I realized good training and compassion was not enough to help some patients, and that sometimes it is necessary to be aggressive and strong when fighting disease and restoring health.

About six months later, a man came to the acupuncture department in a wheelchair. He was in his late 50s and was clearly dissatisfied with life. He came in complaining loudly that he had no faith in Chinese medicine and there was no way it would work for him. He proclaimed that TCM was witchcraft and only good for people stupid enough to believe in it. He ranted, "I have a real disease. I've been paralyzed for more than five years. I've been to the best doctors, Chinese and Western, and done all kinds of physiotherapy but nothing has changed. Nothing has helped before and nothing is going to help now!"

He was very angry and told everyone his son was wasting his time by forcing him to come to this clinic. He continued to disrupt the clinic, but Dr. Lu paid him no attention. She just asked his son for the x-rays and medical history. Then she looked at the man in the wheelchair like she was looking at a small, disobedient child, and told him to be quiet while she needled him or else it would be very painful. The man suddenly stopped talking and looked at her wearily.

As she needled the lines on his scalp, she told him he should be very grateful because, even as loud and obnoxious as he was, his son still cared enough to bring him for treatments. She added electrical stimulation to the scalp and also needled some points on the legs and arms since they were severely atrophied. She then asked him if he thought his son cared for him enough to bring him in every day for the next three months, but she did not wait to hear the answer – she had already moved on to the next patient. As she walked away, she told him to keep quiet because she needed to focus on the other patients.

The man looked shocked at her commands. I doubt many people had spoken to him that way before, and he stayed quiet for the next thirty minutes. After his bell rang and the treatment was over, she removed the e-stim cords and the needles on his limbs but left the scalp needles in place. She told him to stand up and walk at least once around the hospital floor. The man was outraged and started grumbling that it was impossible. She told the son to grab his father's arm and help him up so he could do a lap around the floor because she needed the space for the next patient. She said she did not want to see them again until they had completed the task!

So the obedient son went over to his father and took him by the arm, helped him up and, sure enough, they walked out of the room. Everyone was astonished, mouths wide open, including the other patients and myself, but the doctor said nothing and continued needling other patients.

Even if Dr. Lu's size was not very impressive, the way she talked to people was. In all the time I spent with her, I never saw anyone say "no" to her. It was the way she talked to you. She was very strict but you could clearly feel it came from a place of compassion and understanding.

Five minutes later, the old man came back, drenched in sweat and eyes wide open in disbelief at what he had just done. All he could find to say now was, "I can walk. I just walked!" He sat back down in his wheelchair and the doctor, with a small (almost internal) smile, removed the needles from his scalp and asked him if he would come back tomorrow. He sat stunned, just murmuring that he would definitely come back. And he did, in fact he came every day for treatment and could walk a little further and longer each time. After about 10 weeks of treatment, the doctor told him he only needed to come twice a week, and later reduced that to once a week. In the end, he fully recovered the function of his legs and was walking in the parks every day. Needless to say, his temperament was also completely changed, from an angry old man to a person that appreciated life's every little moment.

Dr. Lu made a strong impression on me and I was able to learn amazing needling techniques from her, but the most important thing I got was that sometimes, to show true compassion to our patients and give them the best care possible, we must be strong or even incredibly strict. She also imparted on me the importance of showing a great level of confidence and courage to guide people back to health. She once said that severely ill people have often lost their pride and confidence, and as their doctor, it was our duty to show them compassion and strength, so they can find it in themselves again.

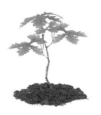

FAITH BUILDING
BY RIKA MIZUNO

Seven years ago, my mother had colon cancer that later spread to her liver. Even after intense chemotherapy and major surgery to remove most of the affected organs, she got sicker and sicker every day. Western medicine could not do anything for the cancer or the unbearable pain without making her unconscious with morphine. Soon after she passed away, I learned about alternative medicine and that acupuncture could have eased my mother's pain. I decided then to study Oriental medicine.

Before I entered acupuncture school in Tokyo, I read several books on Oriental medicine. Many talked about miraculous cures that some acupuncturists had achieved. Reading about these exploits excited me that someday I would be able to do the same. I also assumed my teachers would know all the secrets to health and that my own health would improve just by going to school. Reality was very different. I was shocked to find out that many teachers were actually rather unhealthy and went to biomedical doctors for their health problems. I was confused. It was also a letdown to find out that despite how wonderful our medicine is, it is not easy to make a living as an acupuncturist. I spent the next three years in this state of confusion, but most of my time was spent studying textbooks for the national license exams.

The curriculum at school focused heavily on conceptual material and gave more weight to biomedical concepts. Even after three years of study, I had absolutely no confidence to treat real people, as we were barely given any clinical training with actual patients. Eventually, I decided to go directly into a two-year teacher training program. In Japan, we have to complete an instructor's program to teach at an acupuncture school. But my intention was not to become a teacher, I wanted to gain more confidence in clinical practice. The program offered more practical classes and also an opportunity to work at the school's clinic under the supervision of experienced instructors. It also gave me the opportunity to observe them treat patients.

It did not take long to realize that miraculous cures do not happen often, even for very experienced instructors. No matter how hard I tried, I could not stop myself from thinking I would never really make patients' complaints go away completely. I assumed my clients were coming back just because the clinic charged low prices. I also became aware that our society treats acupuncture as a very minor form of medicine, which most Japanese perceive as painful, expensive, and only good for the aches and pains of older people. I was growing less and less excited about work as an acupuncturist. Of course, I did not expect to cure every patient, and I had not lost faith in the medicine, but my expectations about my new career were changing.

Around that time, I started treating a woman who had pain in her right knee. Treating her would become an incredibly valuable experience for me, one I will never forget. The woman had previously gone to an orthopedist who, although he told her there was nothing wrong with her knee, had prescribed pain medication. She took the pills for a while, but they were not much help and she was hesitant to stay on them much longer. I had treated other patients with bad knees similar to her where there was no apparent signs of inflammation.

In the first treatment, I gave her a simple treatment using typical local points for knee problems with very mild stimulation, just like I had done before and had learned in class. She came back a second time and said she had not felt much change from the treatment. I decided to repeat the same mild treatment since I knew once is often not enough. She came back the following week and told me her pain had actually increased. So in the third treatment, I decided not to needle the painful area directly and instead used distal points on the right leg. She came back the next day and said the pain was even worse! It seemed as if the more I treated, the worse the pain got. She said she had not been doing anything unusual, but now she could not even enjoy her favorite hobby, gardening.

I felt terrible and wondered why she kept coming back to me. On her fourth visit, she finally asked me whether I thought acupuncture might not be good for her. Since Western medicine had not been able to help her, I definitely did not want to give up, so I asked her to give me one more chance.

The situation tested me to try something I had never done before. I decided not to touch her legs at all. I was not entirely sure what I was doing, but I improvised by palpating her back and abdomen. Since she showed some signs that her liver might be affected, I thought her knee pain could be related to the sinews. So, I treated some liver-related points and others that had shown sensitive reactions. She came back the following week and told me her knee pain was about the same. As bad as it may sound, this was actually an improvement as it had been getting worse after every previous treatment. I continued needling in the same style for the next three sessions, and her knee gradually improved until she was pain-free.

The patient herself had no problem with needles, but her legs did not seem to want them. Maybe her pain was related to psychological issues, but in any case the knee itself was not the source of the problem. It was coming from elsewhere. I like to believe that by treating other parts of her body, especially the liver-related points, she subconsciously become aware of the source of the problem and healed it herself. I was so grateful that she did not lose faith in the medicine and somehow was able to trust such an inexperienced acupuncturist. When I look back now, she taught me something very important about Oriental medicine, which makes it completely different from Western medicine. We, as acupuncturists, do not just look at broken body parts and try to fix them. We help stimulate the patients' own healing power by treating them as a whole. In fact, this is what I liked about the medicine and why I became interested in the first place.

Without this experience, I could have remained confused and lost faith in the medicine I had chosen to study. I was so excited at the thought of "curing" people's problems. When I lost confidence in that, I had no idea what to do.

We often do not know much about our own bodies, even though most of our health problems stem from doing things that are not suitable for our body types. The issues will keep coming back until we become aware of these bad habits. As an acupuncturist, I can help people become aware of their bodies, consciously or subconsciously, and thus realize the source of their problems. I was once again very excited that I had chosen this profession. I may not be able to perform miracles, but I can be there to share people's problems and help them believe in their own natural healing power.

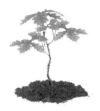

THE ART OF RESISTING
BY GABRIELLE HAMMOND

There is a cosmic joke in the fact that I have two Masters degrees in Chinese medicine. I never intended to acquire even one of those degrees, much less two, and I am privately embarrassed by the replica. Normally people advance in their degrees. I just got the same thing twice. My only solace is this: it represents only that I am forever a student to this medicine no matter how long we have been acquainted.

Lawyer, Diplomat, Ambassador. These were the titles I craved at twenty-two years old. I had been accepted into the American University's School of Foreign Service in Washington D.C. and deferred my enrollment to graduate school for one year to spend time in my hometown of Honolulu to earn some money. College had weathered me and I was a frequent patient of my acupuncturist, a Daoist Master from China who had been my primary practitioner since I was eleven. One day, she asked me to study with her – attend the first class that night. I told her I would never want a practice to treat patients. "You can treat your family and friends," she said. With coaxing, I dropped by the class. I never made it to American University.

I graduated the first time in 1996 from her school in Hawai'i. Under the guidance of my mentor and childhood doctor, I felt homegrown in that environment, safely raised to practice this art. Learning was simple, expectations easily met. When I graduated, I had intended to return to my other ambitions since the four-year program still did not inspire an interest in setting up a practice. But within weeks of graduation, an established and somewhat renowned naturopath who I had never met found me and asked me to join his practice as his acupuncturist. He offered insurance billing, a receptionist, scheduling, forms, herbs, the room and even the décor. I just showed up and treated people. That was the extent of my difficulty in starting a practice: there was none. I was a part of his office for two years, then moved my practice home to share with a fellow acupuncturist a large house with three treatment rooms. It was busy, easy and at times complacent. I did not focus on the business aspect because I maintained another career in nonprofit law for steady income. I worked intuitively and relied on the teachings from my one and only mentor. I didn't have all the answers for everything that walked through my door, and I didn't push myself to. I just enjoyed it. Having only a morsel of luck to tell as my pearl of wisdom for newcomers to the practice, my guess is that the me of back then would not have been asked to contribute to this book.

After six years of practice, I moved from Hawai'i to California for a job opportunity. I casually knew the license to practice would not transfer to my new state, but did not realize this would actually result in having to work at something. I would need to retake almost the whole curriculum in order to sit for the California licensing exam. I figured there were few occupations that improve with age. Medicine was one. I secretly appreciated the break from the pressures and responsibilities of having a practice. Mostly I had no choice. I was not about to let my investment be in vain. Out of loyalty to my former teacher and myself, I returned to the study.

Fast forward through four years of school in a new and more competitive environment: I graduated and was ready to practice in earnest. This time, I actually wanted a practice and I wanted it to be my only career. Truth be told, I wanted a life raft. I had just transitioned out of directing a national nonprofit law organization I had started and grown over seven years. I was leaving a nonprofit law career that had carried me for thirteen years, concurrent with all my acupuncture schooling and practice. The law career had been reliable, demanding, stimulating and ambition-oriented. Now, I had decided it was over. Acupuncture was going to rescue me.

Unfortunately, I felt somewhat mentally crippled within the transition. The study and the demanding job had left me exhausted. While my first school had been grounded in the Daoist philosophy of a particular lineage, my school in California was founded on amassing information. My training left me humbled in the face of so many choices of how to practice, what to practice and in which style. In Los Angeles, healing can be a commodity, not an art. It can cater to celebrities and often demands flash and novelty to be taken seriously. As primary physicians, acupuncturists carry all the responsibilities and liabilities that come with that title, and are expected by patients and medical colleagues to diagnose in both Eastern and Western traditions. After my years of working as an executive, I too had changed. I desired success. I had drive and ambition. I wanted to be the best with a clientèle that validated me.

My mind was filled with tasks and lists that would guarantee perfection – forms I needed to create, promotional materials to generate, billing procedures to articulate, office protocols, treatment plans and business models to write, websites to develop, and on and on. In Hawai'i, my two careers worked to create balance. This time, as I whipped up spreadsheets and documents, I felt rudderless trying to bridge the gap between the kind of practitioner I had been and the kind I thought California required of me. I could not find my pillars of intuition, trust or even comfort. My mind would not shut up. I lacked the ability to slow down.

Nothing quiets you better than immobility. Seemingly without warning, I injured my lower back so severely I could not walk or move. As a person who walked five to twenty miles a day, I suddenly found myself in a wheelchair, unable even to walk the distance from kitchen to bathroom. I rotated through the gamut of practitioners – the best-promoted acupuncturists, physical therapists, chiropractors, energy workers, ayurvedic doctors and massage therapists. Sadly, all without exception misdiagnosed me. Nothing led to even modest improvement. Finally, for the first time in my adult life, I took myself to a doctor. An MRI showed a twenty-millimeter disc had extruded and broken off at L4/L5. This material was sitting on a nerve root that controlled my left leg, threatening to permanently damage it. With a heavy heart and all options exhausted, I accepted surgery.

When the long road to recovery began after the operation, I could not shake the sinking sorrow of feeling let down by my own profession. In my treatments pre- and post-surgery, I encountered practitioners with a wealth of self-promotion and aggrandized certainty of what the problem was and promises to heal it, but they all lacked one thing: care. I did not feel tended to, just placed in the mill of someone's practice. In many instances, their treatments worsened my pain or condition. It was deeply devastating. I questioned whether I would ever return to this medicine again.

Somewhere in my two-year recovery, my life and my mind slowed down. I certainly no longer aspired for a practice built on perfection or high-powered success with a celebrity A list. In fact, I was not sure I aspired for a practice at all. I just wanted life to flow through me and to help my friends and family with this medicine in a manner that supported me and them.

A patient who I had long neglected called periodically to ask when I was going to return to treating. I was a master at stalling on that question, but one day I admitted to her my crisis of confidence in the art itself and my questioning of the whole profession. To that, she said, "If you never stick another needle in someone, I know it is your calling and you have this gift. It was a pleasure to receive that and I'll be ready when you return again." You cannot fight the river that floods through you when someone offers such pure, precious praise. I started treating her mostly out of a strong sense of obligation and silent gratitude for her sincerity.

I did not have much energy, nor did I have any motivation to revisit any of the formerly compulsory lists or business plans. I decided to do what I could and do it as simply as possible. Then there was another friend, another referral and yet another. I saw these few patients in my bedroom, a place completely lacking the professionalism I had hoped to claim in Los Angeles. I diagnosed them using the original philosophy of TCM I learned back in Hawai'i and I did not use the extensive biomedical assessments I had hoped to incorporate. Mostly, I just treated them gently. After they left, I meditated on their health and well-being, and kept a steady focus on my own. Being ill was no longer a liability, but a place that required humility and compassion.

Maybe that is where I had to be to find my own practitioner I could trust. The acupuncturist, whom I continue to see, is a 76-year-old Chinese woman who fills the room with laughter. Her practice is in a dingy old office building that shows all of its twenty years. Her table is uncomfortable, her room cold. But her heart touches me. She gives consistent and thorough care and saw me through that dark period. She does not analyze me and she does not use fancy needling techniques or many needles. She just treats me and treats me well. I promised myself to commit to my own treatments twice a week for two years – regardless of whether I felt I needed it. Going to see her keeps me true to myself and my profession, but more so it keeps me very much in touch with what patients go through – the difficulty of being ill, the little things that become challenges, like scheduling, keeping appointments, prioritizing care and receiving treatment. Her gentle touch inspires me to give the same to others who pass through my doors.

Slowly, with her help, my energy returned and with it my desire to treat more people. I decided I would like to spend time with patients deeply and have time to research things I do not fully understand. I also wanted ample unscheduled time for myself. Writing this in mid-2011, I am eighteen months into my "new" practice. I have a vibrant part-time practice of no more than twenty-five people a week. My patients are from all walks of life, from musicians and actors to teachers and carpenters. Their problems range from common orthopedic pain, to fertility, cancer and chronic disease.

Spending time with a patient last month allowed me to diagnose appendicitis before his primary or even his gastroenterologist did. The patient I am about to see as I write this came in for unspecified thigh pain. Through our work and research, we have just received confirmation that one of the potential diagnoses we had considered originally is correct; she has a pituitary tumor causing Cushing's syndrome. Later today, I will see a patient with multiple myeloma, who for the third blood test in a row is showing improvement. She is off all ten of the medications she was originally on ten months ago for various secondary physical and emotional ailments.

In my practice, I work with some doctors to refer patients and use some biomedical assessments for injuries and diagnoses. I work from a room attached to my home that has been approved by the city as an official place of business. I have my own tax identification number, am listed as a provider with several insurance companies, have a web presence and accept credit cards. I stock a raw herb pharmacy with over one hundred herbs, make my own formulas, make medicinal wines and even grow some herbs. Twenty percent of my patients find me online, thirty percent from insurance company networks and fifty percent from referrals. Somehow all of it was created without a single list or chart.

There are many inspirations in the practice of this medicine, but the thing I draw upon the most is my own deeply cultivated connection to the medicine and its lineage. Primarily, my original mentor from Hawai'i forms a continually growing foundation. She gave me permission to allow for space, not just action, in a treatment plan. With just a little space in and around the treatments, whether doing a meditative art or just giving my mind time to settle, I have been able to notice when something doesn't quite make sense or might need to be investigated. An answer can come, a plan can form. Mostly, I just try to keep myself calm enough to read what is before me.

She is also an active participant in this practice with me because whenever I come to the limits of my knowledge, I put in a psychic request for her guidance. Sometimes, I hear her voice deliver an answer or see her hand needling a point. Of course, when psychic is not good enough, I use the phone.

I have spent a lot of time reading and teaching this medicine. I rely on the academic basics even in the most complex cases. Another teacher, Dr. Zhang, gave me permission for geekdom, which helps my practice immensely. In his mid-50s, with a vibrant practice and an exquisite understanding of herbs, he could be content to know what he knows. But his famous anecdote – comically relayed in his Chinese accent – stays with me:

"Dr. Zhang, you ask, you have fifty years experience. You have twenty patients a day Monday through Saturday. What do you do on Sunday? On Sunday, I study! Always study. That is what my teacher said when he was eighty. That is what I tell you now when I am fifty. Always study."

A smile comes to me when I am reminded of the humility that underscores the service and study of this medicine. And, with that one story, he makes it cool to be a geek and want to read the same books again and again.

Of course, I have practical input. I ask my acupuncturist for her guidance on my patients when needed. There is an email list of practitioners from my California school that hosts numerous treatment questions among colleagues. While I rarely post, I enjoy reading the questions and answers others dialog. It refines my own knowledge.

Currently, my practice is complex and I feel a tremendous responsibility for the people I treat. Thankfully, it also is filled with creativity and insight. I enjoy a mischievous pursuit of learning both during treatments and outside them. I started this journey first and foremost out of deep respect for my mentor. I have been wrong every time about where I thought this medicine would lead me and where it actually did. Today I am deeply grateful for the art of this medicine, its impact on my patients and on me. While I never wanted a practice, I enjoy the one I have now. Maintaining it on a foundation of simplicity, respect and humility is the purest demonstration of gratitude I can offer to those who brought me here. And, it keeps me practicing.

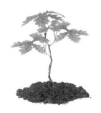

THINGS I DID NOT LEARN
IN ACUPUNCTURE SCHOOL
BY REBECCA PARKER

When I graduated from acupuncture school, I did not really understand the power of what just needles and stillness can do. I expected miracles and I doubted my capability to perform them. My patients have been the ones to teach me how acupuncture works and what they need to allow it to work, and have reinforced my hunch that the process is not about me (or any particular practitioner). Rather, it is about me insofar as how I step back and create the situation a patient needs to heal.

It's not about me

It is my first day at my first real acupuncture job after getting my license and moving back to my hometown. I am sitting in front of my first patient who is smiling in anticipation. She is a regular here at the community acupuncture clinic and has been treated by the other two acupuncturists many times. Now she is actually paying for my green skills.

I am very nervous. My palms are sweating and my hands are shaking. Not as bad as when I had to do thread moxa during my final exam at school, when my supervisor kindly walked out of the room to let me calm down so I would not burn the patient – but bad enough that I feel certain this patient will notice and lose all confidence in me. I have a booked schedule, which means five people this hour, when I am used to treating one in that much time. I am feeling the press of time and this makes me even more anxious.

My patient launches into a complicated medical history involving candida, migraines and many other complaints. Mostly she is bothered by her stomach and digestive distress. I take her pulse and look at her tongue. My mind goes blank. Liver attacking spleen? Spleen qi deficiency? Cold in the stomach? Liver yang rising? As I flail in the quagmire and the clock ticks, one simple thought arises: Dr. Tan's quick-and-dirty digestive treatment. I make my brain search for the image of the flashcard I made with this protocol on it, and start putting in needles. SJ-5, LI-4 and on it goes to yin tang. Pop a few ear needles in. "Are you comfortable like this?" Phew, it's over. The next patient is already sitting down and ready for me.

I felt bad for that first patient, like I had just given my worst treatment ever. I was anxious the rest of the day, but nothing compared to that very first treatment. I will remember it forever. I spent the better part of a year combating feelings of anxiety and uncertainty that this medicine actually works. Slowly, with patient after patient declaring they were improving, I gradually gained confidence. But it was not an easy road. I am not given to hubris or inclined to believe things before I see them. Sure, my patients at the school clinic had seen improvements, but somehow this was different.

Several months later, I found out through someone else that that first patient had proclaimed that day's treatment her best ever. So much for my perceptions of reality. And huh, I guess that Dr. Tan stuff really does work. (Though with more experience, I have found the quick-and-dirty digestive often does not work as advertised.)

My perception is not the same as my patient's. It is not about me.

Create the situation a patient needs to heal

Here is where I contradict myself and say, it is about me, but only in how I make it possible for patients to get better. What patients need is an inviting (culturally, economically, medically) place where they can come as often as they need, where they feel heard and supported, where comfort is paramount so they can go inward during treatment, and where they will want to return.

Trust is a big part of this equation, and this means being able to tell patients when I am uncertain or do not know the answer to a question, or being able to recommend they see someone else with a different skill set. This has nothing to do with needles, and everything to do with how I create a structure and step out of the way.

As many of my patients are new to acupuncture, part of this structure is how I communicate what to expect from treatment. How does it work? How long will it take to see results? Is this or that sensation "normal"? They are building a relationship with acupuncture, and though I happen to be the facilitator, they are the ones walking the path. Actually, we are walking the path together, since as a new practitioner I am also building a relationship with acupuncture, from the other end of the needle.

One thing I never heard much about in school was what to expect during a course of treatment. How long should someone need to come in to see lasting results? In school we were so focused on the points, the diagnosis, the formula, that we neglected the bigger picture of the journey of healing.

I had one patient coming in for Bell's palsy, which he had had for five months. His face was lopsided and he said he missed his smile. He was trying acupuncture out of desperation and was clearly skeptical. He came from fairly far away, and was only making it in once every few weeks. He was not seeing much progress.

Having never treated this condition before, I did some research on prognosis for Bell's palsy and found the consensus was that the patient must come in frequently for quite a while. One source even said thirty to forty treatments would be necessary to clear it up when therapy began a long time after the onset. I had a talk with the patient and we worked it out so he could come in three times a week. After that he started getting results, to the point where he declared himself "amazed" at what acupuncture had done for him. Had I not worked with him to create a better framework for healing, he would not be today referring all his friends and family to our clinic.

Creating the situation where healing can occur was something my first school did well: affordable treatments, a cozy unassuming community clinic, lots of available hours, treating the patients like family, courses of ten treatments recommended. My second school, though amazing for technique, was not so good at creating the right healing conditions. Expensive treatments, restricted hours, a hospital-like treatment room with beds divided by curtains, an expectation among students that someone should be practically fixed in one or two treatments. (I exaggerate, but that is how it felt there, perhaps due to the pedagogical emphasis on one-off grand rounds patients.)

An important part of creating these structures is being a business owner who sets up a sustainable enterprise and manages the systems that make it possible for patients to find me, come to receive acupuncture and get better. I did not learn this in acupuncture school so I am learning it now on my own from the business library, local development corporations, women's empowerment centers and the amazing advisers these places provide.

Given the lack of jobs available for us as graduates, it is unfortunate that we do not at least get a list of resources for this very important part of creating the situation patients need to heal. Learning the Quickbooks accounting software is a lot less tedious when I understand how it will help my patients get better. There are many resources for this aspect of the path to mastery, but one of the best I have found has been the People's Organization of Community Acupuncture. Several volumes could be written on this subject, but I will leave it at that for now.

A patient-centered framework

In the last decade, the Liason Committee on Medical Education of the Association of American Medical Colleges has mandated the inclusion of "cultural competency" education in medical schools, in recognition that a provider's ability to communicate with and gain the trust of a patient can affect clinical outcomes. Acupuncture education holds no such stipulations, but it does not mean that we will not face the same clinical challenges.

It seems there is an assumption that we do not need to learn about the cultural and economic contexts our patients are coming from, either because it is assumed that everyone we treat will be from a similar background, or because of the nature of our medicine. Indeed, we claim to treat the "whole person: body, mind, and spirit." But this definition of holistic is fragmented, as it fails to address questions concerning a patient's place in a societal fabric woven with threads of culture, race, gender, class and other determinants of difference.

Creating the necessary conditions for positive change means stepping out of a practitioner-centered framework and seeing things from the patient's point of view. Asking, "How can I meet my patient where they are?" The Institute for Healthcare Improvement defines patient-centered care as that which "considers patients' cultural traditions, their personal preferences and values, their family situations, and their lifestyles. It makes the patient and their loved ones an integral part of the care team... Patient-centered care puts responsibility for important aspects of self-care and monitoring in the patients' hands... When care is patient centered, unneeded and unwanted services can be reduced."

There has been a lot of talk recently in the acupuncture profession of how we can be seen more on par with medical doctors, through initiatives like the first professional doctorate. But if we really want to keep up with conventional medicine and grow our profession, we would also do well to pay attention to the mainstream trends of intentionally cultivating cultural competency – as terribly cumbersome and inexact as that phrase may be – and moving toward patient-centered care.

For example, I see a lot of transgender patients. Some of them will not go anywhere else but our clinic. This is not always about the affordable prices we charge, but also about the fact that we will not use Chinese medical theory against them. The male/female dichotomy is entrenched in certain yin-yang interpretations. The fact that someone would chose to take hormones or alter the natural physical state of their body willingly through surgery is difficult for many practitioners to grasp. But to create the necessary conditions for care, we must accept the possibility that for some, it is not an option to continue life as the gender they were assigned at birth, whether we can understand or not. Lectures about their liver qi will not help.

But we can be of tremendous help when someone is recovering from surgery by preventing blood stagnation and speeding up healing. We can help when someone wears a binder that makes their shoulders hurt and stagnates their qi. We can help with all the health challenges they might experience just like any other patient, if we just step out of the way, reserve judgment and refrain from asking lots of unnecessary questions only to satisfy our curiosity. In this way, we are creating the necessary conditions for healing to occur.

By creating these necessary conditions, I also create the necessary conditions to get a whole lot of practice. There are two words in this profession I am very partial to: "a practice" is one and "patient" is the other.

Having a practice reminds me that I am constantly practicing. Over and over, with thousands of patients over thousands of hours. My skills are a work in progress and wherever I am right now is just fine, as long as I have created a structure that allows me to constantly grow. I have the tools to help someone in one way or another, but only if I get my baggage out of the way and use what I know, even if it is just a referral out. But I cannot get practice if patients are not coming in, and patients will not come in if the structure they need to heal is not in place.

The word "patient" – although it comes from the Latin meaning "one who suffers" and is looked upon with disfavor by some who feel it takes the power out of the "client's" hands – reminds me that navigating the layers of imbalance toward allostasis most often takes patience, and that time is also one of the elements of healing. Time and appropriate effort are fundamental aspects of mastery and I remind myself of this when I am impatient with my nascent skills.

It is so tempting, when a patient reports good results, to feel powerful, like a wizard who has worked some magic and now gets to bask in the approval of a stranger. But I try to remind myself there are many factors at work, and most of them have to do with things way beyond my control. A midwife I know once replied, when asked how many babies she had delivered, "I have two children, so two." Her point was that women giving birth are the ones delivering the babies. She is just there to catch them and to help create the necessary conditions for a safe birth. To imply otherwise would be to take away from the awesome power of a woman giving birth.

To imply that I am the healer takes away from the awesome power of the body correcting itself. It really is magical, but I did not do that. I just allowed it to happen by creating the necessary conditions, and placing the needles is only a small part of these conditions.

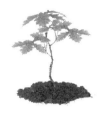

NOURISHING LIFE
BY ELE DENMAN

Lost
Stand still.
The trees ahead and bushes beside you are not lost.
Wherever you are is called Here, and you must treat it as a powerful stranger,
Must ask permission to know it and be known.
...
Stand still. The forest knows
Where you are.
You must let it find you.
       -David Wagoner

It is a quarter to four on a Sunday afternoon in October. I am sitting in the park, a big mug of peppermint tea before me, making revisions to this chapter. Surprisingly, even though it is well into autumn, the sky is blue and the sun's rays are warming me. Gradually I remove my coat, gloves, scarf, and then one jumper and another. I am desperately wishing I had not worn my big furry boots and ski socks! A little boy, wearing only a pair of shorts and trainers, sits on the adjacent bench, noisily sucking an ice-lolly, most of it dripping down his bare chest.

On this mild and sunny day the park is full of families, summer clothes dragged out of the closet for one last outing, and kids are hurtling around enjoying each other and the open space. Over to my left is a small slope and the laughter of the children rolling down the vibrant green grass draws my attention. So much freedom and fun. And I wonder why no adults are joining them in their play. When did we stop listening to the natural urges of life calling us to participate?

The Beginning
Chinese Medicine: This philosophy is new to me. It's fascinating, and it seems to make sense. A way to understand the body as a whole

61

and in relation to the world around us. A way to heal myself, a way to help others. I want to explore it more.

A masters degree program in Acupuncture and Oriental Medicine, in Hawai'i. This is for me.

Three years of full-time study.

Study, study, study – graduate.

Now time for the national examinations.

Study, study, study – pass.

I made it!

I have achieved my goal, and am now ready to set up a clinic and put into practice all I have learned over the past few years. Why do I suddenly feel unprepared?

I want to be as good as my teachers, know as much as them, be able to help my clients as effectively as they can. I want all that NOW.

I feel like a fraud. How can I charge people money when I feel as though I just stepped out of kindergarten?

The Journey

Now begins the true journey. The journey of experience with real clients. This is what will make us as skilled as our teachers, give us access to knowledge and enable us to help our clients in whatever way they need. My journey began suddenly.

Wanting to discuss a business idea that had been evolving as I neared graduation, I invited a dear colleague to lunch at O-Bok, a little Korean restaurant in Manoa Marketplace. The place is a small, simple, old-fashioned diner, and if I had just peered in the window walking by, I would never have walked in. "Service with a smile" was definitely not a concept held in high regard there. But my dear teacher, Dr. Chang, was always recommending O-Bok's cuttlefish soup, and I had finally decided to try it. One mouthful and I was hooked: warming and delicious, I could feel strength and goodness penetrating to my very core. After graduation, it became a familiar place for me and my teacher to visit, where we would share good food and catch up.

And so this was the place I chose to share with my colleague. We ate and afterwards I remember sitting on his balcony, high up overlooking the city. The sun was radiant and light shone off mirrored buildings. I was a little in awe. Not only of the view, but also of my colleague, whom I have a great respect and admiration for. As we talked he announced that he was going to refer all his clients to me when he returned to New York in a few months, and I was stunned.

This man, who had been practicing for more than ten years, was offering me, still a student, his clients. My initial response was to insist I was not good enough or qualified enough, and to say there must surely be a more suitable person than me.

But for some reason, it was me he had chosen, and as I watched the rays of sunshine tracing their splendor over the skyline, I felt honored and appreciative of his offer, and of life itself. I think this opportunity, especially the trust my colleague showed in me, boosted my confidence, and I would draw on this time and time again.

He left the week I graduated in August 2006, and so the following week I stepped straight into a fairly busy practice. Whatever doubts I had or confidence I lacked, people were coming to me for healing. I had to put aside my fears and treat them.

I soon came to realize that even though I was far from a master, I still had something I could offer my clients. I could still make a difference in some way. And in this giving, I received. Each client that trusted me, opened themselves up and was willing to partake in the journey – each gave something back to me and I learned from them all.

I created a tranquil, safe and nourishing treatment space in my home. In every session I gave my very best with the knowledge I had. I held the best of intentions for each individual and I endeavored to remain present for every client. And it was enough. There is something very mysterious and magical about this medicine, this qi we work with as acupuncturists.

Have faith. Do not delay setting up your own practice because of the fear of not being good enough or not knowing enough. Begin your journey and remember, no client turns up at our door by mistake.

> *Something mysteriously formed,*
> *Born before heaven and earth.*
> *In the silence and the void,*
> *Standing alone and unchanging,*
> *Ever present and in motion.*
> *…*
> *Man follows earth.*
> *Earth follows heaven.*
> *Heaven follows the Dao.*
> *Dao follows what is natural.*
> -Dao De Jing, Chapter 25

Presence and Space

After graduation, when starting out as a practitioner, most of us endeavor to utilize the knowledge we have acquired from books, from teachers, from other students, from our clients and from our own personal experience. Our heads crammed full, we try to "do" as much as we can in each treatment; to cause in our clients some kind of positive change to convince them Chinese medicine really works, and to give our treatments validity. We expend so much energy and time trying to "do" – to change, to manipulate – thinking that we know best. But it is actually when we stop trying to do things, when we take a breath, when we step back for a moment to be still and be present, it is in these moments we create a space where there is room for an unfolding, for transformation to occur.

I had the good fortune to study at T'ai Hsuan Foundation College of Acupuncture and Oriental Medicine (now World Medicine Institute) in Hawai'i, under the sixty-fourth Heavenly Daoist master Chang Yi Hsiang, whose lineage and teachings gave great importance to the essence of this medicine.

Coming from England, I can still remember the moment I first arrived in Hawai'i. I stepped off the plane on a Sunday afternoon in August 2003, and was enveloped in a haze of warmth, air heavy with the sweet fragrance of flowers. At the time my head was shaved and as I walked down the steps of the plane, I could feel the trade winds caressing my scalp. Was this the spirit of the islands, the aloha, reaching out to embrace and welcome?

I was full of anticipation and excitement. I had been told someone from the school would come to collect me, and I was secretly hoping they would greet me with a lei.

Almost everywhere I went on the island I could see the ocean. So blue. Sky so blue. Mountains so green. So much beauty to nourish the eyes, to fill the soul. Every day I drank up this beauty and gave thanks. What a gift for my eyes. I thought about people that have never visited the ocean, and instead are greeted every morning by endless concrete tower blocks. What lifts their soul?

There are numerous acupuncture books available and one could spend a lifetime following the directions of these books: what points to needle for certain patterns or symptoms, learning how to measure the exact place the points are found on the body. And in this way one would become a very good technician, following orders and prescriptions exactly. A good technician, but lacking a certain quality, an aliveness.

Alternatively, as my teacher emphasized, one could experience the pure essence of this healing art and see the mystery emerge. One could use the knowledge gained from books, but then tune into each client by seeing, hearing, smelling, listening, feeling and sensing what lies in front of one's eyes; discovering the uniqueness of each individual in that moment. In this way you participate with life itself, you are much more than a technician. You give the very best of yourself. You give presence.

Presence. A consciousness, an awareness, being in the moment, the "now."

Space. Not the absence of objects, not the room we treat in, but an opening, an awareness, a quality we can create and hold in the treatment room, or indeed in any situation.

The qualities of Space and Presence go hand in hand, they overlap. Even though our intellectual knowledge is limited, there is another source of Knowledge we have access to, if only we can be still and witness the present. This is limitless.

> There is a way between voice and presence
> Where information flows.
>
> In disciplined silence it opens.
> With wandering talk it closes.
>   -Rumi

This knowledge, this information, is available all around us, but we have to step into this space of silence to receive it. As acupuncturists, we are taught to balance people's qi; move it when stagnant, replenish it when deficient, and drain it when in excess. If we spend the entire treatment trying to "do" things, we limit ourselves by what we think we know. If we act, and then stand back and be still, observe and be present, we experience the Dao, life itself, the mysterious life-force energy, beautiful, transforming and humble. If we can provide and create space, we can allow it to unfold in its own mysterious way.

This stillness, the space between breaths, is where the transformation occurs, where the seed of potential sprouts, flourishes and blooms.

Qi is the foundation of life itself, the underlying vibration of the universe, making up and supporting all things, differentiated only in density and quality. It is mysterious, with its own intelligence and awareness, which we need to respect and understand. This is what calls us to be humble.

How to define this? Qi? Consciousness? Dao?

> *The Dao that can be told is not the eternal Dao*
> *The name that can be named is not the eternal name*
> *The nameless is the beginning of heaven and earth*
> *The named is the mother of ten thousand things*
> *Ever desireless, one can see the mystery*
> *Ever desiring, one can see the manifestations*
>   -Dao De Jing, Chapter 1

So there is space and there is presence that contribute to the quality of the treatments we give, and these both give rise to Knowledge. These are the elements I have been exploring and delving deeper into since my graduation.

This idea of space was introduced to me just before my graduation. At the time, I was able to grasp the principles and saw glimpses of the experience, but as a new practitioner, my head was full of teachings, the need to cure or heal. Again, the "do" mentality. To stand back and give space brought up fear, of not being in control, of not knowing the outcome. But we must trust. Qi, just like water, knows where to flow. Our bodies are wise and know how to heal. A practitioner can guide the qi, reminding it of its innate natural balance, much like taking the hand of a friend and showing them a new route home. If we walk with them, offering gentle and consistent guidance, they will begin to remember the way. But at some point we must let go and trust their judgment, allow them to walk alone. We do not empower if we are always with them.

I believe clients come to me for this kind of guidance when they have lost the way. My intention is to nourish and strengthen, to empower them so they no longer need me.

As I saw how presence and space were relevant in many aspects of my life, I began to trust them, and myself, a little more. It was a surrender, a letting go of trying to control a situation, and trusting that this force has its own intelligence. I was slowly able to say, "I don't know what will happen, I am not in control." We have a tendency, a need I think, to be seen as in control and knowing everything. But the more we let go and realize we know nothing, the more this mysterious force can unfold. If we can step back, observe and become aware, our treatments become much more subtle and refined, and thereby more effective. It is not that we know nothing, but it is; this is the dichotomy. There is space for both to exist, neither one right or wrong. Both just being.

In the spring of 2007, I joined a Time, Space and Knowledge (TSK) class facilitated by an incredible teacher, Bob Pasternak. I was a little apprehensive as I approached the front door for the first class. I was greeted and led through a delightful wooden house out into the garden. I was introduced to Bob, an unassuming and fragile-looking older man, and I chose a seat directly opposite him on a brightly colored cushion. The sun had already set and the stars were glittering overhead. A glimpse of the full moon rising high into the sky gave me a sense of peace. Or was it the energy that Bob held in that space? Maybe a combination of both.

TSK invites people to explore and stretch their perceptions. We followed guided meditations to consider, investigate and examine our thoughts, ideas and limitations, and how these shaped our reality on a day-to-day level. The concepts we hold often lead us away from a full appreciation of, and participation in, the moment. These are not things we necessarily hold onto consciously, they are embedded in the very nature of our cultural heritage. To recognize these filters, and to learn to exchange them with other ways of knowing, is the exploration we undertook in Bob's classes. The practice in these sessions gave an experiential basis for living consciously in the now.

Bob created a safe space in which to share and explore experiences. He is a great facilitator and healer, and yet remains incredibly humble.

During the time that I attended these sessions, I tried to incorporate the teachings into my acupuncture treatments to investigate their effects. It was a very interesting time for me, exploring the teachings not only in myself, but also in a clinical setting. I began to notice a difference in the quality of the treatments where I actively practiced space and presence, and some of my clients gave very profound conscious feedback, clarifying my own experiences.

One of the exercises we engaged in to explore perceptions of space was relatively easy to play with. Often if we observe stagnation or tension in the body, there is a tendency to focus on the area, narrowing the space around it and then applying some kind of force or stimulation to disperse it. However, if one tries to see the body as space rather than as solid, then the way one perceives the areas of stagnation changes. There is a freeing up, there is room to breathe, to change, to transform. It does not have to be force piled upon force, but an openness that allows a gentle yielding.

Space allows. It is a very subtle thing, and although subtle, this does not mean it is not powerful.

In fact, I have come to believe that the more subtle something is, the more powerful it can be. The more refined a technique, the greater the results, because you are not wasting energy, but doing just enough to initiate the transformation. TSK has enriched my life immensely, and has also aided my development as a healer.

In August 2008, after running a clinical practice for two years in Hawai'i, I returned to England. I had no idea where I was going to live or to practice, only an intention of specializing in paediatrics and studying with a particular teacher. But during a British Acupuncture Council workshop that September, I attended a seminar on Toyohari acupuncture conducted by Stephen Birch. I cannot remember the specific topic of the seminar, but there was something about his treatment style that resonated with me. During the seminar, a volunteer lay on a treatment table. Stephen demonstrated the Toyohari techniques with humor and gentleness, and a deep presence.

Before I knew it, I had signed up for a Toyohari training program beginning the following year, run by Stephen Birch and Junko Ida. The course required me to travel to Amsterdam one weekend a month for the next year – no small commitment. This was not at all what I had planned, but as we all know, life often has its own plans.

So in October 2009, I set off to begin the training, not quite realizing the impact that this was going to have on my practice, and ultimately my life.

I travel to my parents' house in the middle of the night, awaken my kindhearted dad who then drives me to Gatwick Airport at 4 a.m. for my early flight. I am grumpy going through customs, having to remove my coat, cardigan, boots, belt, jewelery and scarf. I decide that next time I will just travel in a bikini and flip flops, and mumble this under my breath as I pass through security.

Easy Jet. Chaotic but cheap. I insert two needles into GB-20 and am asleep before the whole "how to survive a plane crash" demonstration begins. Fifty minutes later I awaken feeling vaguely more human, as the wheels bump down on the runway.

I am in Amsterdam and I am clueless. Which train do I catch? Where is the train? I look at the signs in Dutch and my heart sinks: I don't understand a word. I am definitely out of my comfort zone, feeling lost and insignificant among the crowds of people rushing around with purpose and direction.

But underneath this there is a Knowledge that this is good for me, that it has been too long since I last allowed myself to be open to life. I remember that once you grab the hand of uncertainty and embrace the unknown, not only do you discover parts of your being that surprise you, but you step into a space where incredible things can happen. And I realize I have missed this.

Toyohari is a form of Keiraku Chiryo - Japanese Meridian Therapy. It is a theoretically simple, yet technically sophisticated system of acupuncture. It differs from most other forms of acupuncture in its gentleness, and places great emphasis on the use of pulse diagnosis and palpation.

This style of acupuncture uses "contact" needling (holding a silver needle or probe on the skin without piercing it) and other non-insertive techniques originally developed by blind acupuncturists in Japan. These non-insertive techniques were appealing to me, as I have always been a little needle shy (as my former acupuncture school classmates can surely attest to!).

As the months passed, I realized it was the presence and stillness that emanated from Steve and the other teachers that had drawn me to this style. It was very familiar. It was the same quality I had witnessed studying under Dr. Chang and Bob Pasternak. This, hand-in-hand with a deep humbleness.

In Toyohari, we begin by diagnosing the most deficient meridians (called finding the "sho") and tonifying these. Often, simply tonifying the deficient meridians will balance out any relative excess, eliminating the need to drain or disperse, which could result in some healthy qi leaking out. Toyohari always works to build up the *seiki*, *zheng* qi or "right qi." If your *seiki* is strong then your body can find balance, and is less likely to succumb to pathogens.

There is no need to drain unless absolutely necessary. It is important to always replenish the body, especially in today's society where there is a real lack of nourishment. The intention I hold during my treatments is towards nourishing life. Again, this correlates with the teachings of Dr. Chang, whose treatment philosophy was always to support the healthy qi with the minimum dose, "Less is more."

I loved working in clinic with Dr. Chang. I was like a sponge trying to soak up the ocean of her wisdom. As students, we would sometimes spend twenty minutes questioning a patient before the treatment, making sure we had every single detail of their medical history, present condition, tongue and pulse. Dr. Chang would then come in with a smile, and without looking at anything we had written, lay her hands on the patient at the exact place they were experiencing discomfort.

During a patient's initial treatment, Dr. Chang would use just a few needles, since that might be all the patient needed to stimulate their own energy to return to balance. Her initial herbal prescription would also be gentle. If these proved effective, what would have been accomplished by blasting them with a more potent dose? Not to say this approach does not work, but at what price?

Dose

Amount and intensity are integral parts of treatment. If the initial dose is not enough, you have the opportunity to try something stronger; you can use more needles or a stronger formula. But if you start with your very strongest, you have nowhere to go in subsequent treatments, plus you run the risk of over-treating the patient, possibly even making their condition worse.

This seemed in opposition to many other schools of thought, where a "the more the better" approach seemed the norm. At school some students would question why e-stim was not used, or why cupping or bleeding did not accompany the needles in every treatment, as though we were doing a disservice to patients. The explanation was always the same: The body will get used to the extra stimulus and begin to depend on it for the same initial effect. Over time this depletes the body's *seiki*, its "right qi."

A little nudge might be all that is needed to bring the body's own healing energy back into balance. If required, then of course stronger techniques can be employed, and they often prove extremely effective, but the idea was that they should not be used as a matter of course.

The philosophy of less is more has always sat well with me, and resonated with my own personal experience.

The realm of dose is extremely important in Toyohari also, and administering the correct amount of stimulation requires a high level of sensitivity. The pulse is examined and reassessed after every technique, and the temperature, color and moisture of the body are continually monitored for signs of change. This is especially important when treating children, as their qi moves and changes very quickly, making it very easy to do too much. Any parent would be happier with a small positive change than a big negative one!

As I became more aware of these subtle changes in the body, all of which I now saw as qi communicating with me, I became better at remaining present. If I look or focus too hard, I either end up in my head again, thinking, or miss the signs because my focus is too intense. Like any other skill, the more I practice, the better I get. Sometimes I get caught up in my mind, thinking there is not enough time to look, to observe these new dimensions. But I find that when this happens, it is more important than ever to step into that space, into the moment, and observe.

Spiritual Practice

The final topic I want to share regarding my growth and inner expansion as a person and as a healer, is my spiritual practice. Over the years, a few teachers have shown me the necessity of developing a spiritual practice and of the importance of self-cultivation to become a better healer. My school in Hawai'i emphasized the practice of qi gong for our own development.

In class, we would often recite chapter thirty-three of the Dao De Jing, which embodied one of the fundamental teachings of the school.

Knowing others is wisdom
Knowing the self is enlightenment
Mastering others requires force
Mastering the self requires strength

He who knows he has enough is rich
Perseverance is a sign of willpower
He who stays where he is endures
To die but not to perish is to be eternally present.

I remember one of my first qi gong classes at school: At the altar large wooden statues of Lao Tsu and two Daoist immortals stood tall, the smell of incense filled the air and Dr. Todoki stood dressed in her yellow Daoist robes. Students gathered before her in anticipation, and suddenly a beautiful sound emanated from her very being as she chanted the Dao De Jing in Chinese.

What a sound. I could feel each individual cell in my body respond.

And then it was our turn to repeat the chant. Gosh, what a different noise came struggling out of our mouths! There were a handful of students whose voices projected clearly, and the rest of us mumbled our way through, with me praying no one could hear my warbling. After the chant Dr. Todoki began teaching the graceful flow of the qi gong forms. Chanting was nice, but I decided then and there that my focus would be qi gong.

One visiting teacher suggested we should not worry too much about the effectiveness of our treatments, but to put our focus on our spiritual development, and then when it came time to treat, we would naturally know what to do. This came from a martial arts teacher and healer I had great respect for, but at the time I thought it was a bit of a cop-out. I took it to mean he was saying one did not have to study hard, that there was no need to expand and grow professionally. Now, however, my perceptions have changed and I can understand his words on another level.

The more I can refine and purify myself, the more clarity I will have during treatment. The more conscious I become, the more Knowledge I will receive about the client in front of me, thereby enhancing my treatments. And this does not restrain me from pursuing further education and studies.

Whatever qualities I embrace in my own life, I will of course bring into the treatment room. The more I understand myself, the more balance I create. The more presence and space I acknowledge, the more these will be reflected in my life, including the treatments I give or classes I teach.

For many years now I have maintained a daily qi gong practice. I love getting up when the rest of the world is still sleeping and the sun has yet to rise. The stillness and silence feel magical and are almost palpable. With so few external disturbances, it is much easier to be present. Feeling the air fresh on my face, smelling the morning dew, tasting the salt on the sea breeze, hearing the birds awaken and seeing the first rays of light gently streaking the morning sky: I am filled with a sense of awe as my worries fall away before the mystery and magnificence of life.

My qi gong practice has been through many transformations, and it has kept me sane through the challenges and transitions of life. Upon graduating and leaving T'ai Hsuan, I felt adrift, as though I had lost part of my family. Dr. Ono allowed me to continue participating in the advanced qi gong classes he taught for many, many months, which sustained me until I was able to step away with the realization that I was forever connected to the school, the teachers, and that the teachings were now part of me. This was a great gift.

There have been periods of intense training under gifted teachers or on my own, and times where I have stepped back from the practice for a few days or weeks. And I feel the difference within myself. When practicing every day, I feel small adjustments being made every day to maintain a balance. But after a day or two of not practicing, the lack is distinctly noticeable in my body and in my emotions.

In addition to qi gong, I know I need to sit and be still also. A time to just be, a time to stop, to breathe, to come back to the present. Taking this time has a great impact on the quality of my day. And however subtle, can have an effect on others. I had one client who asked if I meditated before treating her, because she sensed something and would see colors in the morning before her appointment. She had experienced this with other practitioners, but only the ones that would meditate first.

I have a ninety-year-old client, one who I make an exception for with home visits. From the very beginning, every time I placed my hands on her, I got a strong sense of an angelic presence. I felt blessed just to be with her. It took about six months before I had the courage to tell her what I felt. She responded by telling me that every single morning for the past twenty-five years she had been invoking the presence of angels. These experiences validate for me that these subtle practices have an impact and do make a difference.

Everybody will find their own spiritual practice, their own rhythm. There is not one thing that is right for all. But whatever you decide on, I think it is important to incorporate it into your daily life, so it becomes as familiar as brushing your teeth. It is far better to do fifteen minutes every day then to do five hours once a week. It is the constant reminder of coming back to ourselves, of returning to consciousness, of cultivating the qi. The more frequently we can experience this, the greater the impact on our own lives, and thus on the lives of our clients and ultimately the world.

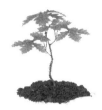

HEN SCRATCHES AND FLY SPECKS
BY R.J. STORM

Now, it should be noted that I really never fit in with the others who decided to pursue the art of acupuncture. Obliged to leave my mountain in upstate New York, I landed in the Big Apple and began an education in medicine and human diversity. New York City. Well, like the T-shirt says, "It ain't Kansas." The college I went to was filled with a cross-section of people from many walks of life and everyone had a past more unique than the next. Massage therapists, contractors, artists, former military, some young and some beyond middle age, many colors and many talents. But here we all were, rallying around the common goal of helping people.

Each individual who pursues acupuncture, no doubt, has a story of how they chose this path and became aware of the benefits of acupuncture. I am no different, I have a story as well. First off, I am a farmer at the core. Nobody special, just a working schlub who grew up shoveling dung, bailing hay and sawing wood. Humble beginnings to be sure, and the only privileges I had growing up was the inestimable value of hard work and learning to shoulder responsibility at a young age... not a typical background among my contemporaries.

The propinquitous environment of acu school did grant me an unmatched opportunity to develop skills to meet the unique demands of working with different types of people in school, as well as the diverse patient base of a clinic in New York City. My God! This was the first time in my life I saw a form that said, in all sincerity: male, female, other. Back where I come from, the checking of "other" meant someone had a problem, but even alluding to this fact was certain to raise the ire of one or two of my classmates, who would staunchly demand, "Are you trying to pathologize this?" What? No, I only submit that these people are somehow a quarter bubble off plumb, and at very least are worthy of note in the record. After all, the fact has been deemed worthy of inclusion on the intake form.

It has always been difficult for me to accept the extremely casual way many practitioners dress. Starched, white lab coats covered shirts left untucked, wrinkled clothes and a general carefree attitude toward personal appearance. Personally, I favored a shirt and tie. Not that I thought myself better than anyone else, but to establish trust with new patients, I thought it seemly to put my "best foot forward," as my grandma had admonished me a million times before. And at least at that time in the student clinic, it seemed to fit. I never want to make the poor feel poorer in their own eyes by the clothes I wear, but this is not a small Chinese village, and let's face it, most people in America have certain expectations of a medical professional.

And the kooky music in American acupuncture clinics, what's with that?! The "breathy," Yanni-like, synthesized, pasteurized, homogenized music that goes on and on, round and round, like some rudderless dirigible puttering around in the uppermost reaches of the ozone layer. What ever happened to regular music? Personally, I like my music the way god intended it to be played: bluegrass style. But I admit that can be taxing for some people. In my own practice, I keep a CD player around and let my patients bring their own music, or I have a laptop available for them to choose music from Pandora.

Anybody practicing sees all kinds of people, and ideally you should be able to connect on some level with anyone who comes through your door. That being said, I think it is natural to develop preferences for certain types of patients, and to be realistic about who you can and cannot connect with enough to build that all important rapport.

But in all seriousness, I went to a great college with a lot of great people who resonated with many types of patients. Me? I just happen to resonate with the working class. The mighty multitude of folks who get up every day, step up to the plate and swing the bat. And as long as you get on base, you done good. Some days you smack one over the fence, some days you only tap a nubber up the third base line for a single, other days you might draw a walk... and occasionally you get hit in the head with a pitch... but you got on base! Ya done good.

Somewhere midway through college, I heard more than my share of "When I was in China..." So, after finishing school, I went to live in China. In fact, although my beautiful Chinese wife and I go back and forth, we consider China our home. Working short-term contracts in the city gave me the chance to work in small rural villages. A local authority in Yichuan, Henan Province, made me a village doctor. They figured if a crazy American really wanted to come to a place with no heat in the winter and no running water at anytime, and still wanted to see 100 patients every day... go ahead.

Yichuan is, after all, where my wife is originally from. I had to travel 10,000 miles to meet the girl next door. And I traveled 10,000 miles to meet some of the richest people on Earth. Good people. People who work hard and learn to shoulder responsibility at a young age. People who sleep with a contentment not of this world. And so many of these people smoke! A testament to the human condition. My father-in-law – baba – is an old farmer and house builder. Today, like many from the villages, he goes to the big cities to build tall buildings. But the truly amazing fact is, like many rural Chinese living simple lives, he smokes three packs of cigarettes a day and maintains a blood pressure of 106 over 68. This, of course, does not mean his lungs are in good shape, but it does bear eloquent testimony to the marvelous multi-redundant compensative mechanisms of the human body.

Speaking of cigarettes, many patients at my village practice were sent home with the following instructions for heat therapy between visits: Use the business end of a cigarette to apply heat to deficient points. And this is no doubt the healthiest thing a cigarette has ever been used for. Since it was a foregone conclusion that nobody was going to stop smoking by their own initiative, it became clear that the healthiest thing a cigarette could do would be to heat prescribed points. Not exactly TCM protocol, but this is China. Patients with difficulty talking fought a constant battle with plum-pit qi. These people often saw stellar results with twenty tobacco "ouchies" bilaterally at SP6 every day. While the heat source is not exactly a beneficial herb, the tonifying properties of injecting heat into deficient points got undeniable results, often within a week.

Married to a great woman who is also a farmer at heart, I got a chance to fully immerse myself in Chinese culture. I loved learning classical Chinese medicine. There is nothing like schmoozing with twelfth generation acupuncture doobies, people who have to get results in a land with few medical options even in emergencies. So, for the rest of my life, I will pick up what tidbits I can from the old guys who have really studied the classical texts. I can then go back to America, get on the college lecture circuit, shamelessly pander my manuscripts, and preface each talk with, "When I was in China..."

Few people in China like pain. Few people anywhere like pain. That whole *de qi* sensation can be brutal and if you want to repel people from your doors, it can work wonders. For some, this feeling is an integral part of treatment, but in the style I practice, *de qi* seems to be quite unnecessary to obtain measurable and immediate change. A Chinese villager, having spent a life exposed to the raw elements, can have skin that is half-tanned by age thirty. I vividly recall, on more than a few occasions, using .018mm x 30mm needles with an insertion tube at points such as LI10, SP6 and especially SP4, the needle would simply bounce right off the skin... several times. Often large moxa balls were required in the winter months to clear diagnostic reflexes and effect change.

Simple heat therapies achieved astounding results in a variety of complaints: ST13 for prolapsed uterus, LV5 for enlarged prostate, LV8 for fibroids or certain tumors, etc. Musing on these results, perhaps one reason is that Chinese villagers' bodies are primed for health owing to their simple diets with very little meat, plenty of exercise, drinking nothing but water and tea, and getting a good eight hours of restful sleep. I observe similar, but slower, results in the USA, but the same results as in China can be achieved easily if an American patient makes a few lifestyle changes to parallel their Chinese counterparts. I do not know anyone in America who gets eight hours of sleep, restful or otherwise.

It was a big question in school to figure out what exactly to say when a patient asks, "So, how does acupuncture work?" I try to avoid just putting in the standard tape and pressing play, but the general answer I use goes something like this:

"Acupuncture is an ancient form of treatment with roots that go back many thousands of years. Acupuncture deals with the concept of qi, which, according to the Chinese physiology, is the ethereal life-giving energy that circulates through our bodies. However, qi does not circulate arbitrarily, but rather through definite pathways called channels. Therefore, acupuncturists don't just put needles arbitrarily into a person's body, we put them into points on these channels. All together, there are about 400 points we learn in school. With these, we access the body's qi to drain away things that are in excess, strengthen things that are deficient and move things that are stuck. After you learn what the points do and where they are, you learn how to decide on a palate or a constellation of several points suited to a particular patient to restore the balance of qi and bring about health. That being said, let me remind you that the name is Storm, not Christ, so if you're looking for miracles you should be in church. Any questions?"

Humor is an important part of a practice. I recall taking practice management classes back in school and listening to what seemed like a pedantic nattering metaphysical French philosopher from the 1500s who was drunk on cheap wine. Here in America, at Storm's Poke 'Em and Smoke 'Em Clinic, we see an endless parade of characters. And far from delicate Oriental statuary and paintings, the place is adorned with guitar, banjo, mandolin, Dobro, some fiddles and a big old bass. Afternoons sometimes turn into jam sessions, with the instruments changing depending on who is on the treatment table. I never wanted to be spa person, just a country doctor who makes people feel better so they can get to work the next day and deal with the occasional emergency. The professional and serious side is there, but I feel humor should be often injected to keep things light. Even if someone announces they have the "Big C," you can always look straight in their eyes and remind them this is not the 1500s, and today a lot of people have whipped cancer and gone on to gloat about it for years to come. In fact, entire gloating clubs have been formed!

My basic policy is if a person doesn't feel better when they leave than when they came in, they don't pay. Fifty beans ain't going to make or break me, and people should see something for their money. I decided a while ago not to be greedy. Better to take less and see more people, and to avoid making acupuncture prohibitive to the very people that need it. One of my intakes may go something like this:

R.J. - And headaches?
Patient - No
R - Unusual sweating?
P - No
R - Ever had a kidney stone?
P - No
R - Would you like one?
P - ...???... NO!
    ....we laugh.

Often, prior to moxibustion, I plead with a huge manly man on the table – manlier even than me – to tell me when they feel the point get hot. It is surprising how many will not say a word during a treatment, but complain to their wives how hot it was. But I have found I can always get a response by telling them, "Look, there are no extra points for martyrdom! Our policy here is warm bodies in, warm bodies out. The neighbors have their eye on the clinic. And visits by the ambulance – or worse yet a hearse – are bad for business. So please, when it gets hot, say 'hot!'"

And hours, I like to sleep late. In bed by 3 a.m. and try to start the day by noon. For me, this works. Suppose you are a single parent who opted not to shake down Uncle Sam. You have no health insurance and work two jobs. For you, coming in at 2 p.m. or during the day on a precious day off is tantamount to giving away a tooth. But these people can often make it in at midnight or 1 a.m. I treat a lot of people at night. And, having gone without health insurance, been in debt up to my eyeballs and scared to peek in the mailbox lest I have to face some fresh horror from a heartless relentless tyrant of a collection agency, I never want to become so arrogant as to forget what that feels like.

It seems that many people suffer a similar plight with, sadly, more to come as the decay of Western civilization continues. The two big thieves of the medical arts – probably society in general – seem to be apathetic complacency and complacent apathy. These eat into our vitals and rob us of our joy. And daily vigilance is necessary to guard against the corrosive effects of unchecked mediocrity. In its stead, we must unleash our genuine desire to do the right thing, seek the honorable path, raise up the standards of humanity and be anxiously concerned with the ones we treat. Only then will we be worthy of calling ourselves practitioners of a healing art. This is clearly not the time to assume an adversarial position of "us" and "them", it is a golden time to enlarge the "us" and shrink the "them" so eventually there is only "we."

In conclusion, let me add that all acupuncturists use needles, but not all needle users are acupuncturists.

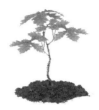

THE UNEXPECTED ROLLER COASTER
BY IAN STONES

I guess the best place to start is to tell you a little about myself and how I came to be an acupuncturist. After all, there are not many people who grow up saying they want to go into acupuncture. I was never hugely academic at school but I did ok. I got through my GCSEs fine and went on to do my A levels. These, however, did not go so well, as I never really applied myself. College was not the thing for me and I had no idea what I really wanted to do. I had an interest in the technical aspect of theater production and music, and as a guitarist I enjoyed playing in a band for many years. But unlike those who know they want to be a doctor as soon as they are out of nappies, I never had any huge urges when it came to a career.

My elder brother had gotten into lifeguarding, and I followed suit, as there was an easy route in thanks to him. Initially I worked part-time at a sports center as a kids' party organizer and then later as a lifeguard. I soon became full-time and moved on to duty manager and lifeguard/first-aid trainer. It was not particularly what I wanted to do, but it seemed a natural progression from where I was.

I was around the age of eighteen and still working in the sports center when a friend of mine expressed an interest in the fire service, so we visited his local retained station. I really enjoyed it and wondered if there might be similar opportunities in my hometown of Yateley. I popped down to the station and was added to the waiting list. Some two years later I was finally invited for interview and eventually accepted as a retained firefighter. The retained fire service was a great starting place for me and helped develop my interest in the service as a full-time career. As a retained firefighter I was on call when at home or within easy reach of the station. I soon learned to live with a pager permanently attached, and to drop whatever I was doing when it went off.

As I built experience in the retained service I decided to make it a full-time career and started applying to different brigades in the area. I faced several challenges; not only was I very nearly too short, although fit and healthy I was also too young and lacked the life experience the fire service requires. Nevertheless I was eventually accepted into the Ministry of Defence Fire Service. So at last I was sorted, a full-time firefighter for my career and a retained firefighter in my off hours.

Unfortunately, the full-time station I was posted to had been buzzing with rumors of closure for some time. I soon heard of an opportunity at a nearby soon-to-be private airport, so I made inquiries and without too much effort was offered a place. At the tender age of twenty-four I settled into a new career at Farnborough International Airport. To some extent it was great, as I had a good income and most of it was disposable as I was still living with the folks. I started saving for a house and was just generally enjoying life. However, after a year or so I started to feel bored and restless. I was working 15-hour shifts with very little to do. I did get to enjoy my yoga, guitar and reading while at work, but with so much time to kill and stuck in one place, it got very tedious.

Over a period of several months I became more and more restless. I loved the retained fire service since it was more like a hobby, but the full-time job was dull. By this time I had discovered acupuncture through treatment for hay fever. I loved chatting to my practitioner and hearing about Chinese medicine, and it was through these conversations that I came to attend an open day at the College of Integrated Chinese Medicine in Reading. Having been inspired by my visit, there was no stopping me. I was so amazed by acupuncture that in October 2003 I handed in my notice at the airport and went off to study acupuncture, funded by the savings I had set aside to buy a home.

As I write this, it is nearly seven years since I made the leap into studying acupuncture, and now aged thirty-three it is just over four years since I graduated. I will never forget those last few days at college, revved up and ready to get started. I felt it was time to get out of school and start my own practice. Many people are nervous at this stage, worrying about the lack of supervision, but I could not wait. I was hugely excited about my new career and starting to see patients.

However, graduation did come with a certain awareness of the challenges that lay ahead. Having worked as a lifeguard instructor and within the fire service for a number of years I had been through the ups and downs of developing new skills and building confidence. With acupuncture, I knew this was just the beginning of my career and I was fully expecting to face difficulties; this I certainly did, but not in the areas I was expecting.

I went into my studies through a need to do more with my life. My interest in acupuncture reared up when I felt the urge for a career change. Did I really think about long-term goals and realistic career/life outcomes? Probably not, I was only twenty-six at the time. I wanted a change and something new, so I approached study with the attitude, "I'm sure I'll enjoy it and it'll be a worthwhile experience no matter what."

I did and it was. College was excellent, and I was enthralled by all we learned. I did well throughout the course, made some special friends and was pleased with my final grade. I remember one day doing the math in my head trying to establish what I could earn, "Ten patients at £38 a treatment, not too bad for a few hours work. This'll be great." Maybe this is where the problems started.

In May 2007 I was set free and was in the fortunate position of being able to join my current practitioner in her practice, with a room available pretty much as and when I needed it. The treatment rooms were part of her shop on a busy main road. She had been there for ten years and had a reasonably busy practice. I started like many with the odd patient here and there. I treated friends and family, and the other practitioner passed the occasional patient my way. In the meantime, I juggled a few of my previous jobs and hobbies, including lifeguarding and first-aid training. The retained fire service had remained a constant even from the days when I left the airport and was still stimulating me and providing an income.

Within a couple of months of starting, I received a call from a practitioner I had observed when I was a student. She was leaving a multi-disciplinary clinic nearby so she could practice from home, and offered me the opportunity to take over her slots. This was fantastic news for me, as she was fully booked several weeks in advance. I thought this could be the greatest of opportunities, so I took it.

So here I was with two practices and still working as a retained firefighter. Things were looking good. I planned to build the two practices and in time I would leave the retained fire service behind and concentrate on acupuncture. Fantastic! All seemed rosy as I had no major financial burdens. But as time went on, the vision of what I wanted to achieve began disappearing. I was struggling to get new patients, and having taken over at the multidisciplinary clinic, I realized the majority of patients follow the practitioner they were seeing before or just stop coming.

With just one or two clients a week, my interest and enthusiasm were beginning to wane, and the prospect of acupuncture providing an adequate income seemed rather unlikely. This was probably my first minor blip. It was early days though. I was still only a year or so in and I knew this was going to take time, so I was not overly hard on myself. I just thought I needed to do something about it, so with some half-cocked ideas and renewed enthusiasm, I set off on a minor marketing campaign. I went around to local businesses making sure I had leaflets out and paid for some advertising space in different local magazines and newsletters. Of course this all had to be funded from my low acupuncture income. The efforts were to no avail; very few patients were coming. No problem I thought, just stick with it.

Over many months, things gradually began to pick up in the multidisciplinary clinic, and I was now returning to a reasonable position. A good week would see around six to eight patients and a quiet week three or four. My confidence was growing, and this was a huge help in managing my patients and feeling good about what I was doing.

By now I had also become involved with the professional body in the U.K., working as part of the office team looking after the acupuncture student community. This was a great job, as it kept me up to date with the profession and I gained a lot of experience in talking to the public about acupuncture. The other benefit was that I could help students progress in their new career and my experience would influence the way this happened. I got to meet lots of students and share their concerns and worries.

I have found there is an amazing optimism in the student community. They are keen to learn and love what they are doing. It is not like I do not remember those days, after all they were not that long ago, but following my recent struggles I look back with slightly less of the rose-tinted view most students seem to have. Meeting new students is part of my job, and I sometimes wonder if they have done their research properly and realize just what they are heading into. Of course, it would be unfair of me to say anything on their first day, but I do recommend they think about how they will start their business.

Meanwhile, as time plodded on it became apparent things were not working out with my two practices. Over the period of a few months, I left my original practice and joined a new chiropractic clinic in Farnham, having considered several different options en route. The new chiropractic clinic seemed like a really good opportunity. It was a fresh start and I was the sole acupuncturist. By now I had a reasonably full diary one evening a week at the multidisciplinary clinic and things were definitely on the up. The chiro clinic came with its own unique set of challenges, but has taught me a huge amount.

For one, I knew how weak I had been when it came to dealing with patients and getting them to commit to treatment. I cannot say whether all chiropractors are strong marketers and business people, but those at this particular clinic certainly were, and it worked in my favor. The chiro clinic started just as the others, with the odd patient here and there, but the clinic owner worked hard at promoting me and business grew reasonably quickly.

I still had the vision in my head of two busy practices, but it was slow coming. Then, out of the blue, the owner of the multidisciplinary clinic informed me he was pulling the plug. I was stunned, but had mixed emotions about it. Part of me was pleased, as it meant I was no longer running between practices. That was countered with disappointment, as I felt I was just beginning to make it work there. However, I was also relieved that I did not have to keep struggling to make it work. This was a strange thing to admit to myself, and made me wonder how much I really wanted this. Still, I was now in a position to put all my energy into one clinic, which was a first for me.

So what has the roller coaster ride been like? I would say in the early days it was all about coping with next to no patients. Initially this was ok. I could accept this was going to be the case. I did not come out of college expecting to be busy within a few months, but I did have the impression I would be busier than I was. Nonetheless, I had the odd moment where I felt really low. Around two years after qualifying, I started to question what I was doing; not necessarily my treatments, but my career choice. This seemed to be far harder than I thought and I was not seeing the money I had hoped for. I was surprised when this started to rustle up feelings of resentment about my choice. I began to feel I was owed a profession. I should be making a decent living out of this. Why isn't it working for me? Why can't I get new patients? But I soldiered on. I just accepted this was something I had to go through, and in time it would all work out.

In September 2008, a year and a half after I qualified, I went on a study trip to China. This was one of the greatest things I have done. I met some great people and it revitalized my practice in the short-term. But by the following September, I hit my biggest low of all. This was when I seriously considered walking away from acupuncture altogether. At this point I was only in the chiro clinic. Things had not been too bad, but my plan was always to get to around thirty patients a week to make a comfortable living, and this just did not seem to be coming my way. I hit a quiet couple of months and was feeling hugely disheartened. Not only was I asking the same questions as before, but I now began to question acupuncture itself. Did it really work? Did I believe in it? This was huge to me. It began to undo everything I had worked so hard for.

On top of all this I was feeling the financial pressure. By now I was living on my own in a rented flat. I was still working with the retained fire service and the British Acupuncture Council, but it was a struggle. It bothered me that I did not have a pension, I could not afford to buy a house, and even a holiday seemed out of the question. What sort of a future would I have if this was the way it was going to be? It was at this point I started making tentative inquires about going back into the fire service full-time. But when I found there were no opportunities, I decided this had to be the time to make acupuncture work. I was not going to let this beat me. I had invested too much money and time to just walk away. I owed it to myself to know that I had tried everything.

Over a couple of months I worked on a new website and again invested in marketing my practice, this time with a little more focus. Business picked up and I had several patients pay for a course of treatment up front, which is always a huge boost. Before long I was back on top of my game. One day saw ten patients in the diary and they all showed up. It was a pleasurable trip to the bank that week.

This sort of day would send me to the absolute opposite end of the emotional spectrum. Why would I want to be employed? This is great. I'm earning good money in just a couple of days a week. I'm my own boss and I love it. My patients appear to be doing well and they all give positive feedback. Yes I still have a part-time office job, but that complements my private practice as it is still involved with acupuncture. All is great and I'm happy.

So what happened next? Well, the roller coaster continued and I was starting to find the ride a little tedious. It would seem that what goes up comes back down. My busy period was followed by another very quiet month and I went right back at questioning myself. Except I had realized the questions are even bigger and far deeper than before.

I began thinking about the whole work-life balance. It seems acupuncture ticks so many boxes for me: the freedom of being my own boss, the love of what I do, the positive results my patients experience. But I have also seen the other side of the coin, which is the financial insecurity, the non-stop challenge of running your own business, the lack of pension or future security. My main question seems to be about what I want from my work. Do I want to do something I love but is a near constant struggle, or should I look for a less fulfilling job that pays a good salary and affords me a better quality of life?

It has been quite a revelation facing these questions. I really was not expecting to find myself in this position, but I am sure many other people go through similar things. The outcome can only be down to each individual, as all our circumstances are so very different. The practitioner who has finished their full-time career and practices as a "hobby" will have a very different outlook than someone like me. I had no idea what I was getting myself into with this and only now realize what a huge learning curve it has been.

I did some reading about career changes and attended a very informative marketing seminar. At the marketing seminar, everyone had to say where they were with their business and where they wanted to be. I figured, let's be honest, and I told the group I had serious concerns about my long-term future and how difficult it was to run such a business. This was met with what felt like a great wave of comfort from the others in the room. Everyone seemed to have faced this battle, and even practitioners of twenty years experience explained that they struggle with the roller coaster income. This was great for me, not because I came out with all the answers to my problems, but because I knew I was not the only one and I was not being unfair to myself.

I must say I have felt a little animosity towards the profession at times; if only I had really understood the challenges that were coming. It is easy to lose yourself in the wonders of Chinese medicine when starting out, but for those wanting to make a living, you have to realistically think about your future, not just hope the universe will provide. Unfortunately you do need to consider how you will pay the mortgage, whether you can afford to pay into a pension, and what will you do when it is quiet? I feel that realistic outcomes and expectations get somewhat glossed over, and it would be nice to see this change. I think new graduates need to be armed with a whole set of skills to face the challenges and realities of starting out.

It seems the tide is beginning to turn in this respect, and teaching institutions are putting more emphasis on the importance of marketing and promotion. My role within the professional body has allowed me to bring some of my personal issues into the services new graduates are offered. A business support program is now available to help people in the early days of practice, and I am hoping to launch a supervision-style workshop to support those with under five years in practice.

I would like to see even more honesty within the profession about what lies after graduation, so practitioners are fully prepared to build their practices and achieve the success they hope for. If I am not the only one who has been through such experiences, why are we all not being more open about the difficulties we face?

On a personal level, the last few years have made me examine closely what makes me tick. It seems I have a restless nature and need constant stimulation, but I fear that changing careers again would only lead me down another path where I get bored after a few years. Do I just accept this or do I try and find a way to deal with it? My current acupuncturist says I need a job that keeps me busy and offers me variety. Acupuncture does do this to a certain extent, but it does not appear to offer the stability I want. It would seem I want to have my cake and eat it too. Is this too much to ask from life?

My advice to anyone considering making acupuncture a full-time career is to think about the things I have had to ask myself. Your position may be completely different from mine, but realistic expectations are a must. I, like many others, fell in love with acupuncture and the astounding mystery of Chinese medicine. I now have some amazing knowledge, skills and experiences that will never leave me, but I am in danger of disregarding these because of my business expectations being shattered by a very harsh reality. Those who can afford to go into this profession as a sideline or just to earn a bit of pocket money are onto a winner. My advice to people who want to make it a full-time career is to be sure of what you are doing, have a plan and really commit to what you want to achieve. Do your research and make sure your expectations are realistic.

I have no doubt there are hundreds, if not thousands, of practitioners who have succeeded, in fact I have met many of them. Is it luck of the draw? Right place right time? Is it all about having a good business head or previous marketing experience? Who knows, but it can be done and I wish anyone and everyone the best of luck with their practice.

For me, maybe it was my restless nature or maybe it was trying to start a practice in the middle of a recession. It could be any number of things, but it has been an invaluable learning experience so far, and I look forward to finding an answer one day. Over the last couple of months I have had a major shift in my expectations that has made me feel far more comfortable with what I can achieve. I may never get to practice acupuncture full time, and although I would like more stability, the money I earn is not too bad. But maybe I am on the up part of the roller coaster – who knows what is around the corner.

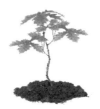

ON BECOMING
A COMMUNITY ACUPUNCTURIST
BY PAMELA O'MALLEY CHANG

Sometime in the last month – the third anniversary of opening my clinic and 3½ years since obtaining my acupuncture license – I realized I had finally become comfortable with being a community acupuncturist in a high-volume, low-fee clinic. More important, my clients are comfortable enough to consistently fill my twelve scheduled hours per week with fifty-plus appointments. Reaching this point has been a gradual and cumulative process, but it is a far step from my student expectations of having a patient load of maybe five cases a week.

In school, although I liked the intern clinic and had several regular clients, I did not expect to continue to practice acupuncture, except perhaps as a hobby. First, I did not think I would find an entry-level acupuncture job in my vicinity. Second, I was afraid of opening my own practice – scared mostly of cost, for both me and my clients. I could not imagine seeing more than one or two clients per hour, and I could not see covering my overhead and making a profit without charging $50 to $100 per treatment – a price I was not comfortable either paying or asking my friends to pay regularly or long-term. Fortunately, half a year before finishing my internship, I learned about the community acupuncture (CA) practice model. In community clinics, one acupuncturist treats several clients who are seated together in one large room. Treating four or more clients per hour allows the acupuncturist to charge fees as low as $15 per visit, yet still gross $60 to $100 per hour. Suddenly, I saw a way for me to have an acupuncture career.

Within weeks, I enrolled in a workshop called "The Nuts and Bolts of Community Acupuncture" sponsored by Working Class Acupuncture (WCA), pioneers of the CA movement in the United States. WCA generously shared the systems they had developed for running a high-volume, low-fee acupuncture practice. They showed us their open-seating treatment space, described their sliding-scale fee structure, demonstrated five-minute intakes, taught *jingei* pulse diagnosis for rapid assessment of which meridians to treat, and even outlined an "invisible receptionist" system for acupuncturists without office staff. Moreover, WCA had set up the Community Acupuncture Network (CAN, now absorbed into a multi-stakeholder cooperative, POCA – People's Organization of Community Acupuncture), an on-line forum for sharing information about opening and operating community clinics.

Attracting and keeping a clientèle, I think, is the biggest obstacle new practitioners face. WCA's template gave me a ready-made business plan, one that had already proven its success.

Immediately after graduation, I started meeting with two potential business partners. We spent six months talking, visiting other community clinics, shaping our common vision, looking at places to rent, researching, making lists and creating budgets. Eventually, a pattern emerged: one of my potential partners kept seeing obstacles; the other did her homework, got things done, and cared about launching a CA practice more than she feared the future. In the next two months, between late January and mid-March 2008, Tatyana Ryevzina and I settled on a business name, wrote our partnership agreement, rented and furnished our clinic space, obtained business licenses and permits, and opened Sarana Community Acupuncture in Albany, California. The vision of offering affordable acupuncture in a safe and comfortable group treatment area, becoming a first-line resource for the ordinary health needs of our community, and creating a fulfilling workplace gave us a clear sense of purpose. We run our business because it shapes the world we want to exist.

From opening day onward, we attracted enough clients to meet our monthly expenses. In our first month, we were open twelve hours a week and typically saw between twenty and thirty clients per week. Gradually, we added shifts. Now we are open 41 hours per week and four acupuncturists see about 160 clients each week. None of us earns much, but we all get reliable paychecks.

As a new acupuncturist, the first thing I struggled with was becoming comfortable as a clinician. This was difficult for me even though I had been relatively confident in school. Some of my confidence came from being older than most of my fellow students and from having felt success in prior careers. More of it came from my experience as a TCM patient. In my second year of school, I was diagnosed with stage-1 ovarian cancer. Opting for TCM over chemotherapy, I experienced the process of gradually rebuilding my health by getting weekly acupuncture, boiling raw herbs, taking herbal-extract powders and pills, renewing my qi gong practice, altering my diet, and taking time for adequate rest. By the time I began my internship, I had received acupuncture from several competent clinicians and had made many of the lifestyle changes I would be recommending to my clients. More, I knew what to expect from TCM treatment and I knew that it had worked for me. Nevertheless, during the first few months in my own clinic, being an acupuncturist seemed like a performance. I felt my clients were watching me and I had to act as if I knew what I was doing. I needed to have answers when clients asked me what I saw in their tongues, why I put that needle there or what I felt in their pulses.

Gradually, experience accustomed me to the role. I developed my stock phrases: "The tongue is the window to the internal organs," or "That point's on the same meridian as your problem." Once, caught in a moment of utter candor, I replied that feeling pulses was just something I did while I decided what points to treat. I learned that this answer sufficed and that saying "I don't know" did not lessen my patients' trust in me.

Still, even when I regularly got instant results from the Master Tung points recommended for headache (ST-36, beside ST-36, and GB-34), I did not feel I was a "healer." I did not feel I had the "magic fingers" one of my classmates seemed to possess in her instant ability to find sensitive *ashi* points. But one day, after I had been practicing for nearly a year, one of my clients burst into tears during her intake. In silence, I passed her the box of tissues, stepped back while she composed herself, then inserted her needles. She slept, awoke in better spirits, went home and wrote me a thank-you note.

I realized then that my gift for healing is in holding a space where people can feel safe and acknowledged. I can listen to them and bear witness of their struggles. I do not have magic fingers, but it does not matter. My job is to be as trustworthy and caring as I am capable of and then to step aside. In fact, the longer I practice, the less I think of myself as a healer. I put needles in; I pull needles out. Maybe the most effective thing I do is drape blankets, tucking people in for a cozy nap. People heal themselves – or not. The most I do is to set the stage.

The other thing that was hard for me as a new practitioner was developing speed. One of my strengths as a clinician is my ability to listen. In school, this meant the talkative patients found their way to me, yet these were the clients who were most exhausting. CA appealed to me, in part, because it precluded much talk. But how was I to transition from treating one patient per hour to treating one every ten minutes? Because I did not know any better, I made a gradual transition. For my first two months, I scheduled appointments at twenty-minute intervals, then at fifteen-minute intervals for the next year. Then for another six months, I scheduled five clients per hour. For the past eighteen months, I have been scheduling six patients per hour and sometimes treating more. By contrast, my most recent colleague at Sarana began scheduling six clients per hour immediately. By this time, of course, we had trained our clients to need little talk, and had created lists of point protocols for the most common ailments and a file box of point recipes for less common illnesses.

During my first year or so, I always felt rushed and behind schedule. Much of my time was consumed in talk. It took a long time for me to recognize that the more I spoke, the more people got caught up in wanting to talk about themselves. I had to learn ways to avoid triggering long conversations – like asking, "What can I treat you for today?" instead of the open-ended, "How are you?" I had to learn to interrupt the history of an injury with the request, "Can you point to where you feel the most pain now?" More, I had to learn to trust that I could create an effective acupuncture treatment knowing only the chief complaint, pulse and tongue.

Many people helped me streamline my intake process. My business partner, with five years seniority over me as an acupuncturist and one year seniority as a community-style practitioner, was my foremost instructor. Tatyana gently nudged me to assert myself and set boundaries for patients, like the "qi hog" who consistently arrived during my lunch hour, then talked for twenty minutes (at least) before settling in for treatment. Tatyana also shared her Master Tung point prescriptions and outlined the script all of us now follow for new-patient orientation and intake.

The CAN forum provided other tips, the most useful of which was the recommendation to stop taking notes during intakes. When I put the clipboard down, it felt as if a wall between me and the patient had disappeared. Our conversations were no longer interrupted while I wrote things down. I could think about what I was hearing *as* I heard it. This meant that instead of waiting until the end of the intake to review my notes and then select treatment points, I could tentatively choose points throughout the conversation, and modify or discard them as the intake progressed. Of course, this grasping at treatment points before having a *zang-fu* diagnosis was diametrically opposed to what I was taught in school. But Richard Tan's "Balance Method" seminars had already shown me that a *zang-fu* diagnosis was not the only way to practice acupuncture.

Finally, my patients are my ultimate teachers. They show me that acupuncture works: sometimes instantaneously, more often gradually and cumulatively, sometimes spectacularly, and sometimes not well enough. Many of my clients come week after week for months or even years. Their regular attendance means we develop a comfortable, ordinary relationship. In our five-minute conversations, they tell me of their aches, pains and challenges; of births, deaths and everyday stress. They see me on days when the clinic runs smoothly and on days when I am running late. They know me well enough to tell me such things as: "your hands are cold," "you forgot to take my pulse," or, "you need to stop and breathe." (Whereupon I did and thanked the client.)

The ordinariness of our relationship takes the pressure off me. I do not need to have magic fingers or expert answers; I am just an ordinary person – albeit with specialized knowledge – doing what I can to make people feel better. I do not have to agonize over selecting the perfect point prescription; I can try balance method one time and *zang-fu* treatment the next, and have the patient report back which worked best. Often it turns out that both treatments are effective. Thus, my patients confirm for me the CAN dictum: "Frequency always trumps modality." That is, how often people get acupuncture is more important than what specific points are selected.

In these three years, I have become comfortable as a community acupuncturist and my image of what an acupuncturist is has evolved. I no longer get anxious when two people are waiting to be treated and two more walk in the door. I have come to know, as CAN-founder Lisa Rohleder pointed out in her keynote address to the 2011 CA Conference, that for community practitioners, acupuncture is not primarily a one-to-one interaction. Instead, the primary relation is between ourselves and the treatment space, whether it holds two, nine or twenty occupants. We work the room as a waiter works a restaurant, trying to give everyone a satisfactory experience.

And that satisfaction is not solely our creation. We provide the opportunity, but our clients bring expectations, willingness to share naptime with others, and participation in maintaining a peaceful, healing space. I have learned that I am a server, not a healer, and it is the community of all of us together who make the clinic a success.

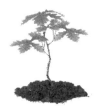

A FRESH LOOK AT OUR ANCIENT ART
BY HIDENORI TOMITA

Japan is one of the few countries with a long history of Oriental medicine. Despite these rich traditions and a wealth of unique techniques, the acupuncture market in my country has been seriously depressed for several decades. According to statistics I have seen, only seven percent of the Japanese population has experienced acupuncture. Adding further stress to this paltry state of affairs, there are more than 140,000 licensed practitioners in the country and 4,000 new acupuncture graduates needing to make a living every year. I have spoken to an accountant who said eighty percent of acupuncture clinics go out of business within three years, meaning people lose not only their jobs, but the opportunity to practice and improve their skills. Even in such a severe environment, I left a secure career in marketing to explore the potential of acupuncture.

My first experience with acupuncture was when I was studying at a university in Honolulu. At the time, I knew nothing about Oriental medicine, even though I had spent the first eighteen years of my life in Japan.

I had started having severe back pain and I had visited several doctors, but got no relief. A good friend recommended I go to see Keiji Inuo, a veteran Japanese acupuncturist who has lived in Hawaiʻi for years. Under his care I got better quickly. The results he achieved impressed me and sparked my interest in acupuncture. Even after I was cured, I would visit his clinic to study with him or to share a bottle of something nice to drink after he closed the clinic for the day.

After I returned to Japan, I got a job at a giant advertising firm, but going back to school for an acupuncture degree was always in the back of my mind. Working for a big company was a little boring, but I did learn about marketing and business, which has helped me run my clinic. In Japan, acupuncture is not really considered part of the medical field, it is more of a service industry. Unfortunately, acupuncture schools do not offer any business classes, so graduates are professionals but not businesspeople.

There seems to be two main reasons Japanese people do not choose to receive acupuncture. One is that a lot of them have negative preconceptions about acupuncture – they think it will be painful or are scared of being burned by moxa. Others see it as superstitious or related to some kind of sketchy religion. There is a serious lack of knowledge of and experience with Oriental medicine. Cost is the other big reason. With national health insurance, almost everybody can afford to go to the doctor whenever they want. But if you want acupuncture, you have to pay for it completely out of your own pocket. Most patients, indeed most consumers, are pretty smart with their money and the level of satisfaction they demand has been rising. If we can get people to believe the benefits they receive from acupuncture exceed the price they have to pay, they will flock to our clinics.

At the same time, I have found that most people are subconsciously curious about acupuncture. When I am out drinking and people discover that I am an acupuncturist, they are really drawn to the topic and ask lots of questions. So there is a deep-down interest, but people need an extra push to actually make an appointment. I believe that people in our busy society have huge stress levels – both physically and mentally – and acupuncture can be a solution for them in many ways. Since we practitioners already know this, we just need to convince the public that acupuncture can be an attractive alternative to regular doctors.

With the biggest challenge being getting people into the clinic, I have worked very hard in making mine as attractive as possible. From my experience in marketing, I knew good aesthetic design is an essential part of business success. Most practitioners just focus on their needling skills, and neglect the atmosphere of their clinic or the message they are sending to the public. Many of my colleagues run their clinics from a room in their homes, and it ends up looking like a part of their living space. We do not go into other people's homes very much in Japan, so it is difficult for patients to be comfortable in such places. I believe design not only involves an object's appearance, but sends a message about what a particular business values and offers.

My small clinic is historical in its look, recalling the style that was common in the Tokyo (then called Edo) of two-hundred years ago. I tried to achieve the peace and grace of a traditional tea house, letting the natural quality of the construction speak for itself. My treatment style is also based on classical acupuncture. I wanted both my treatments and the setting I provide them in to reflect a traditional, simple beauty – to be an oasis for my patients. Actually, some people come to my clinic for the first time more out of interest in historical structures than a desire for acupuncture.

I tried to imbue all aspects of my business with this traditional, simple beauty. One patient said that after seeing the style of my website, he thought I might be able to see his health problems in a different light than medical doctors or conventional acupuncture practitioners. My design concept extends to music, and my patients listen to traditional Chinese music during treatment. I have heard that clinics in the West play soothing music in the treatment room, but for Japan, this is quite unconventional. I think a lot of people, especially the younger crowd, do not choose acupuncture because most clinics lack creativity. Japan has many skilled practitioners, but they lack imagination, especially outside the treatment room.

I feel it is important to get the word out about what I am doing. A lot of people are scared not only of getting acupuncture, but are uncertain about what type of people practice acupuncture. I try to make use of modern media as much as possible – writing a blog, using Twitter, publishing a web magazine and holding small events at my clinic. My blog gets several hundred hits a day and I write about a variety of things, from how Oriental medicine can be used in daily life to what is going on with me personally. Most patients who come to my clinic say they read my blog before making an appointment to see what kind of person I am.

I realize most patients do not come to acupuncture clinics just for relief from physical pain. They are usually seeking other benefits from treatment. If we cannot meet their needs, they may as well just go to a hospital (at least in Japan, where we have universal health care). One of the most important things patients are looking for in a traditional practitioner is communication. A common complaint about going to see a regular doctor is that the examination only lasts five minutes after you have waited for three hours. So providing time for proper communication is a very important part of what I do. This extends to aftercare as well, such as emailing patients to check on how they felt after the treatment. I try to convey that I am their personal acupuncturist and they can contact me anytime they feel in need of help. I think good communication can improve the effect of the treatments, and I feel really happy when a patient says they think of me as their family doctor.

With these efforts, my patient numbers have been increasing, even though I charge the going rate in Tokyo, about sixty dollars a session. I think this is because my patients get more for their money seeing me than going to typical acupuncturists. If we show the public we have original solutions to their problems and our services are an excellent value for their money, people who have never experienced acupuncture will pay attention, and interest in our traditional medicine will grow. I hope the day will come when people think of the neighborhood acupuncture clinic as a place to go for their everyday health problems.

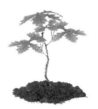

A COMPLETE 180... OR NOT
BY DAVID VITELLO

Things were changing and I needed help. Being a middle-class guy from New Jersey, the last place I expected to find myself was with some Korean massage therapist at my local yoga studio. But there was no other place to go. My life was changing – my physical, psychoemotional and spiritual dimensions were way out of balance, nothing made sense anymore and life felt hollow. Friends and family no longer comforted my current concerns and conventional medicine had nothing helpful to say about my digestive problems, circulatory issues and stress levels.

So there I was, lying face-up on a massage table, experiencing my first massage, just hoping to relax a little bit. The practitioner was a short Korean man with the most gentle and kind temperament. He had been teaching the qi gong classes I had started going to in the morning.

After doing some regular bodywork on various areas, he started doing Chi Nei Tsang abdominal massage. Very quickly my entire body started buzzing intensely. At one point I opened my eyes and saw him waving his arms above my abdomen and I began sobbing uncontrollably. Watching him work, the feeling got more intense. Thoughts raced through my mind, "Wow, there really is magic in the world. How is he doing this? What's going on? I'm really being healed somehow." I let go of a lot and cried for the rest of the treatment. I left asking, "What the hell was that!?" But something had happened, a shift, an experience that would guide me inevitably in a new direction.

For about a week after that treatment, I was different. I would get emotional for no reason, I walked slower, and the world seemed clearer and more beautiful. It was a completely different way of experiencing life, which had previously been filled with rushing around, getting things done and no real awareness of my surroundings or other people.

I had not been seeing this amazing thing called life: it had been reduced to a series of tasks.

I experienced this bodily buzzing and emotional release a few more times. I visited another healer that did laser acupuncture. It was a weird experience overall, but when I lay on her table and she began asking questions and doing intuitive work, it happened again. I got Chi Nei Tsang about a year later and it happened again. I also did a session of Stanley Grof work, where you do rapid deep breathing to send the body-mind into an altered state, and had a similar experience. I continued to have these releases, and I believed they were therapeutic.

Prior to all this, I had been working a tech job in Phoenix, was in a long-term relationship and did the usual things a 27-year-old does, I guess: working and hanging out with friends and my partner. But after three years at the job, things shifted dramatically. The relationship ended, work seemed pointless, the repetition of the lifestyle I had lived throughout my twenties became stale and I developed some heath issues. Life just did not make sense any more; a change in my relationship to life was necessary. Everything indicated that things simply were not working anymore. This was a painful time, but also filled with excitement for discovering new values and interests. I went to that massage to relax, hoping for just a little help, but what I experienced was a shift in my perception of reality and life, and I knew it would never be the same.

Along with these efforts to heal and the transformation of my consciousness, I had been bitten by what some call the "enlightenment bug." A search had begun for deeper meaning, real experience and connection with Spirit (whatever that was). I also wanted to engage in a profession that mattered. Looking back, I can see now that I simply followed in the footsteps of previous generations, looking to the East and its spirituality and medicine for answers. I was filled with immature preconceptions about what enlightenment was, what Oriental medicine was and how it would all be, which is never what we find in reality.

But why get involved in some foreign medical practice that sticks people with needles and prescribes odd medicinals that are supposed to restore "balance"? What are we all looking for when we begin our exploration of this medicine? I believe most Western students come into it looking to connect with the depths of life, which have largely been washed out of our modern world of rationality, science and reductionism. This drive to connect with life on a richer level is exemplified by the culture of the 1960s and 1970s, when a major shift took place – from modern rationality to postmodern pluralism. Old values were transcended and new ways of being and making sense of life emerged in that generation. Interest in multiculturalism, relativism, altered states of consciousness and Eastern spirituality replaced the view of the world as a well-oiled machine with natural laws that could be learned, mastered, and manipulated for one's own purposes.

When one enters new territory, it is a time of great excitement and possibility, but it is often infused with unconscious projections and idealism. There are so many ideas about what these new interests will provide, about how correct and better they are than previous understandings, or how they will solve all our problems. But these beliefs are immature projections. After investing a few years or decades exploring the landscape, our idealism drops away as we are faced with the complexities life and the failing of our attempts to make sense of it all.

In my case, this initial infatuation and process of superimposing romanticized concepts and ideas onto Oriental medicine and the ancient realized Daoist masters who supposedly created it lasted about two years. At first this new world seemed quite magical, so beyond the way I had been making sense of reality. But I learned quickly that the ideas I had of a super-spiritual medicine from the East that could counter all the negativity of my own culture was simply wishful thinking. As I probed deeper, I saw contradicting concepts, the vast theoretical literature of the classics, and most notably that this medicine is subtle in nature and not as clinically superior as I had hoped.

Scholar vs. Practitioner

A central dichotomy in most fields is the tension between conceptual frameworks and real-world application. As humans, we have a need to give meaning to our experience. But how well do the conceptual structures we build help with all the complexities and unknowns of the real world?

The simple fact is, as any expert in any field will tell you, when one probes deeper, the questions get more complex and plentiful. From quantum physics to inner phenomenological explorations, in the end we have very little we can rely on conceptually that brings us to comfortable and lasting conclusions. If anything, concepts provide temporary stories we can use to communicate our experiences, but they never really say it all. The old adage: Try explaining how chocolate tastes to someone who has never had it. No words or concepts will suffice. I certainly do not dismiss intellectual endeavors and the need for accurate conceptual models, but I bring up this point to dispel the notion that any one perspective or framework holds the complete truth and has the final word.

A balance of scholarship and clinical experience is optimal, but most people tend to be drawn to one side rather than the other. There are some Oriental medicine practitioners who tilt to the theoretical and scholastic side of our profession. They are often incredibly adept at the Chinese language, translation, classical sourcing, Asian culture and the like. It seems these types value the Chinese classics and history, and are apprehensive about modern interpretations and creative alterations.

This is a beautiful side of the medicine, but in my opinion should not be allowed to stunt the clinical exploration of Oriental medicine in the West. By all means, those interested in these aspects should pursue it with utmost energy, as this will help all Western practitioners learn more about the roots of our medicine.

The other extreme of this polarity can be seen in the clinician who abandons all classical theory as nonsense, and reinterprets acupuncture and herbology to fit whatever their current worldview may be. Some new-age practitioners, for instance, create their own metaphors and ways of working with energy to fit their postmodern worldviews. Or there are the creative types who are always trying to come up with something new and groundbreaking that puts them on the Oriental medical map. These types value creativity, modern interpretations of the classics or biomedical explanations, and struggle with the clinical relevance of vague and contradictory traditional material.

I try to value both approaches and to see their positive contributions and shortcomings. I believe each camp is at its best when it is healthily balancing the other polarity's tendency for pathology. Stagnation and fundamentalism can be countered by creativity and modernization, or uninformed reinterpretation and reductionism can be countered by classical mastery and further translation of the Chinese medical literature. I believe our perspectives need to hold both of these realities in a dynamic play, instead of picking a side and defending it.

Much of my earlier career seemed to revolve around a search for the "best" way to practice. Sure we are told about the harmonious plurality of Oriental medicine and the wealth of styles available to practice, but deep inside I always thought there must be a superior way. This is probably a very Western ideal. Looking back, this search had other motives besides the simple desire to be a good practitioner. It was a search for secrets – the special points and herbs that would not only heal my patients, but provide me with professional notoriety and material success. I was looking for the true medicine, spiritual medicine, the right medicine, all fueled by an underlying desire for self-preservation, success and, of course, to be an exceptional healer.

I sought out a "spiritual" school for my education that taught Daoist medicine in addition to traditional Chinese medicine. I tried to absorb as much as possible from the school's founder, following her around, competing for space in her clinic, trying to make a connection. On the surface, all of this was to be a good healer, but those less-than-noble underlying motivations were there too. It was actually quite painful at times, to see the neediness of a hungry ghost seeking information and teachings in myself and others.

This teacher gave extraordinary explanations, used points for spiritual indications like resolving karma, and applied special herbs, formulations, charms and Chinese astrology in her treatments. She seemed to practice a unique mixture of TCM and shamanic Daoism. This was a very difficult time for me, as I was trying to determine if this was what I was interested in, if this style was actually more efficacious than other approaches, and if this was indeed the spirituality I had envisioned and come seeking. It seemed a stark contrast to the Buddhist meditation I was practicing and connecting with, which was based on ideas of egolessness, fundamental awareness and compassion.

I finished my masters degree there, maintaining an open mind and steady practice of the school's lineage qi gong style. By the time I graduated, I was very much into spending an hour with a patient talking, then needling, then doing some qi gong therapy mostly from an institutional standpoint. I enjoyed connecting with patients at this level but always felt a bit doubtful and was never completely convinced I was doing them any good. Some reported positive results and seeing white light, while others seemed uncomfortable and skeptical.

I believe there is nothing more beautiful than putting your hands on another human being with the genuine intention to help them in whatever way is needed at that moment. Through breath and compassion, letting yourself and your agenda to be there completely with the pure intention of healing is truly special. On the other hand, I can think of nothing more narcissistic than someone with a Jesus complex who is using the encounter to show off their special qi powers, in effect making the entire healing situation about themselves, consciously or not. It is tricky stuff and requires impeccable honesty and integrity.

After graduation I did a complete 180. I moved to Seattle and met a wide variety of acupuncturists, one of whom inspires me to this day. I went to her with some of my spiritual treatments and ideas from school, looking to show off my knowledge, and she simply said, "Results. It's all for nothing without results." A fancy conceptual theory means little if it amounts to nothing in the clinic. She never condemned my explanations or what I had been taught, but simply showed me what worked for her and emphasized she only cared about results. She practiced a style of acupuncture that focused on palpation, trigger points, motor points and more modern ideas on acupuncture, but she always included some TCM or meridian theory in her treatments. She had a busy practice and I felt something very genuine about her. She was a true healer and not just acting like one or preaching some fancy spiritual philosophy.

I stopped practicing qi gong soon after the move to Seattle. I became even more involved in sitting meditation and the Vajrayana energetic practices of my teacher's lineage. While this practice deepened, my qi gong practice faded. I started feeling silly about moving my arms around, and my initial ideas about teaching faded quickly. I was now on to the exploration of biomedical acupuncture, trigger points and the like. And for the first time, I felt like I had found a way to practice that matched my temperament and worldview. Mystical Daoist explanations and the search for secret points and styles no longer interested me. Rational explanations and the physicality of trigger points under my fingers was my new direction. However, I continued to practice meditation daily and met my root teacher, so my spiritual interests were still very strong.

For the next four years I delved into the work of Mark Seem, Alon Marcus, Matt Callison, Shudo Denmei and Jason Roberts, all of whom spoke of the importance of palpation, trigger points, meridian-based acupuncture and tender spots. I largely dropped the use of TCM acupuncture and patterns, although I still use this system for a small portion of patients. I began focusing on meridian-style treatments and the release of holding patterns in fascia and muscles. Most importantly, I started to see results. Not amazing or magical by any means, but there was a fairly big difference between what I had seen with purely TCM acupuncture and patterns.

Taking the Magic Out of Life

In the last year, I have begun teaching at an acupuncture college and have greatly enjoyed it. I have had the opportunity to teach a biomedical course on anatomy and physiology, as well as an advanced TCM course on nephrology. There is a striking difference in these topics and the reactions of students toward them.

Biomedicine with its scientific basis leaves very little open for the average anatomy and physiology student. There is a basic core of material to be memorized and very little, if any, of it speaks to the multiple levels of human existence (matter, bioenergy, mind, spirit). This reductionist worldview breaks everything down into physical constituents that interact mechanically to produce a human, and is based on the classical Newtonian ideas on matter and energy, of solid individual bodies moving predictably in empty space. Western medicine is further influenced by the Cartesian view of the body as separate from the mind or soul. Viewing the body as a machine and the mind as the commander is a product of the industrial-technological-social system of the last couple of hundred years. Just as the Chinese used waterways to make sense of their bodies, the West used the machine metaphor. More modern, but nonetheless incapable of accurately reflecting the true complexity of being human.

I personally highly value biomedicine and the amazing amount of exploration it makes possible at the molecular level, but it always seems very conceptual and far from real experience. We do not experience neurotransmitters and synapses firing, we feel sensations and ride the waves of quickly fluctuating experience.

In contrast, during Oriental medicine classes students always seem more alive. There is a sense of wonder, new possibilities and creativity. The deeper layers of human existence are relevant and of high importance in Oriental medicine. Bioenergy, qi, life force, sensation, breath – however you want to conceptualize it – is a central concept, and the influence of psychological and emotional states on disease is basic theory. The connection of man to spirit and nature is a central theme in both the classical literature and clinical practice. There is much more room for conversation about deeper questions, levels of experience and life.

Acknowledging the many dimensions of being as a part of our ancestral understanding is a central concept in most traditional healing systems. This is the reason students in our field still have a glint in their eye, a heart open to possibilities and a soul that sees magic in the world.

There has been no reduction or denial of the unknown. The students are not bogged down by a neat conceptual framework that reduces experience to physicality and only that which can be seen. They are interested and inspired to explore unseen bioenergy, the soul and spirit, which holds enough inspiration for a lifetime of work. In this realm, life is much more than pieces of matter bouncing off each other in space. It is relational, sacred and magical, with concepts failing to justify its complexity and beauty.

I often find myself teetering the edge of both worlds – wanting science to embrace and genuinely investigate the subtle aspects of human experience, while also wishing complimentary medicine could be more scientific and efficacious.

I practiced for four years in Seattle. I did not open my own clinic because I knew I would be moving out of the state sooner rather than later, so I worked with chiropractors and part-time at a busy acupuncture clinic. I was able to work full-time as an acupuncturist after about a year and a half, and after four years was earning about $60,000. Most of the time, I was working fifty hours a week, six days a week, at four different locations.

It was never as stable as I wanted it to be and I never had the desire to work that many hours. Being employed at small businesses had it ups and down, but when it comes to stability, it is definitely down. If things were slow, my hours and patients got cut. My early dreams of working a few days a week and making $100,000 a year seemed so foolish. In all honesty, I did not feel I could raise a family on that income, and the instability and amount of overtime presented other obstacles. Eventually, I began exploring the idea of becoming a nurse practitioner, seeing this as a way to secure nine-to-five work with benefits and a middle-class income, and also something where I could keep practicing acupuncture and herbal medicine to some extent.

The next thing I knew, we were off to Honolulu and I was applying for the University of Hawai'i's masters program in nursing and my wife for a masters in social work. I felt I had given Seattle all I had. It had been a great place to practice and afforded me many opportunities for learning and clinical growth.

After moving back to Hawai'i, I spent a year teaching at my alma mater. Teaching has been a wonderful experience and it is so true that you learn the most when you teach. I have really enjoyed scouring through texts trying to put together good classes. I also supervise at the school's student clinic which, more than anything, has been challenging and insightful.

There are so many conflicting emotions and views that pop up when we are forced to step out of our cozy conceptual caves. I see students grasping desperately for a TCM diagnosis, thinking if they get it just right, the patient will completely recover. I have been there and I know that is often not the case. Healing is so much more complex than a TCM pattern. There are others who have a natural ability to connect with patients, yet struggle to find words or Chinese medical theories to describe it. Some do not want to be challenged at all, they just want to be right. They have no interest in learning and evolving because they cannot let their guard down enough to be open to something new. And I see others who are afflicted with a poverty mentality. No matter what they are told or do, it is not enough. They will continue to take CEUs and expend untold energy trying to find "The Best Way." There are those who search for magical points and spiritual treatments, others who pray or do qi gong healing. There are endless ways of attempting to heal a patient, and endless attempts to feel good about the method one chooses to use. It is beautiful and complex, as is everything.

As with most things in life, I am left with more awe and openness than anything very useful to say about how things should be, or what is right or wrong. Our medicine seems so complex and metaphysical that any conceptual story is doomed to fail to contain it. But of course I have my preferences, as we all do and should. So I am off to get a bio-medical degree in hopes it will enable me to practice integrative medicine and have a stable career that will support a family. I hope to practice acupuncture and herbal medicine in a Western clinic where I have the ability to order blood work, labs and medications as necessary. I am excited to see the differences between the people attending the nursing program and the students that study Oriental medicine. Will they be dismissive of qi, organic food and meditation? Will they be into mainstream culture, cling to reductionist outlooks, McDonald's and Costco versus farmers markets, new-age spirituality and energy?

I think I will find more of the same in most respects: people searching for meaning, stability and wanting to do some good in the world. That eternal striving for happiness, comfort and safety. These always make their way into whatever we do, be it waving our hands to clear stagnant qi or prescribing a pill for diabetes. Our actions are informed by our struggle to exist in the way we believe we should, or have been told we should.

But what if we let go of those desires? What if we put aside the need to be happy, safe or right? Let go of the ongoing struggle to be someone special, smart, a healer, a classical acupuncturist, a success. What if we stop our quest, be nobody, and settle right into our present experience without the slightest resistance? Doing that may bring us a healing that is of the deepest nature, even if its for only five minutes a day. This has been my true passion since the beginning, since the bug bit me, and this continues to be my primary calling. The thing is, now I know I do not have to be a "Chinese" medical practitioner to live it, I can be anything... and no-thing.

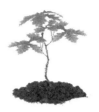

WORK IN PROGRESS
BY BOWEN WEI

When I sat down to write this essay about my experiences as a recently graduated acupuncturist, I realized it would mean sharing the history of my life with the reader. This is because destiny did not lead me early on to be an acupuncturist. In fact, I find I am still having a hard time living up to this title. But as I thought about things, I discovered there were key events that helped shape my view and approach to the healing art I try to practice. My life is a constant work in progress, the "here and now" seems just an illusion, and talking about the future makes God laugh; but I am thankful for the chance to stop and ponder who I am.

My name is Bowen. I am forty-eight years old. I was born in Tokyo and lived there until age sixteen when my mother allowed me to leave the family. I moved to the United States alone, the year John Lennon was shot.

Without the protection and guidance of any elders, my path has not been straight. There have been many crossroads in my life. My childhood dream of becoming an architect went up in smoke with the first joint I was offered. Instead, I enrolled in art school, studied photography and ended up working odd jobs. Those years, my twenties, were emotionally challenging. I was not the happiest child to begin with and, maybe because of this, I had a series of encounters with people who had been emotionally and physically abused, one of whom I married.

By the time I was twenty-eight, I was so unhappy I decided I needed to find the seed of my misery. One night I had a dream: I was trapped in a small, dark octagonal room with eight doors. I opened them one by one, but there were only brick walls behind each one. Out of desperation I looked up, and there was a beam of light!

I delved into my past and traced a lot of my suffering back to an unhappy event that happened at age five. I made a journey back to Japan to communicate with my siblings who had harmed me. In the end, their initial response did not really matter. It was the beginning of resolution and reconciliation. Peace took many more years, but finally it came.

With my personal life back in some semblance of order, the next step was to get my professional life in line. In many ways, I owe my life to the man who showed me the ropes as a graphic artist in New York. It was my first "real" job. Not only did he teach me the importance of asking for appropriate compensation for my work, but he helped me develop skills that are valued in any field – an eye for detail and the patience to perfect.

As I slowly become financially flush and began to feel the sense of power that comes with this, I lost my moral rudder. I wanted to hurt another by way of rejection, just like had been done to me. The abused became the abuser.

A few years later I moved to Hawai'i and fell in love with life outside a city. I experienced for the first time the immensity of the ocean and the generosity of mother earth. I learned immediately that to be with nature is to be humble. Having been taken down a peg, I recalled a story from one of Carlos Castaneda's books about the teachings of Don Juan. Before beginning his studies to become a sorcerer, Don Juan asked Castaneda to make an inventory of his past and to offer a sincere apology to anyone he had ever hurt, no matter how small the deed. My journey as a healer started then, almost eighteen years ago.

As beautiful as Hawai'i is, I was never able to stay put for long before itching to move. From 1997 to 2003 I was continuously on the road, seeing the world, flying, meeting, creating... and falling again. This time it was not another I hurt, but myself. I was playing the role of owner-chef at a restaurant in Brazil, being creative and making new friends. I partied too hard thinking the end of the world was coming, but then it didn't. It was a very psychedelic time and I truly believed I had seen aliens.

But no trip to outer space came, only depression. To clean up my chemically altered body and soul I traveled to Thailand and spent four months receiving massage and acupuncture, and I began learning yoga and meditation. Coming back to Asia after twenty years in the West was for me a positive awakening. In the Buddhist presence of Southeast

Asia, I felt I regained my balance. I returned to Hawai'i, continued studying massage, got licensed, and found work in a resort spa and also alongside a few chiropractors.

Things seemed to be going well, but then I began working with a group of acupuncturists, and I suddenly felt inferior. They spoke with such certainty, they made sense and they did less physically demanding work. So against the opinion of a good friend, who pointed out that I would make better money as a massage therapist, I eventually quit my jobs, moved to another island and enrolled in acupuncture school. Almost as soon as I began the program, I realized how much of the foundational knowledge of TCM is woven into Japanese culture. It was refreshing but familiar at the same time. For example, "*Genki desu ka?*" (Japanese for "How are you?") is quite literally "How is your *yuan* qi?"

No matter if it is visual, culinary or healing, for me being an artist is all about offering an experience. Money or income potential is never my first concern when I start a new project. The process has always been more important than the outcome. And I have always been able let my creations go once I reach a certain level of satisfaction. (This is why I do not consider myself conventionally successful, but that is another story.)

An artist's job is to provoke a desired emotion in their subjects. This provocation comes from knowing the rules, but purposely throwing things off balance. In the healing arts, I believe, the job is not about removing a symptom (leave that to the M.D.'s, whose subjects must be "patient") but to lead the client to the cause, to truth. Ultimately, everyone wants to be happy, but ignorance leads to self-abuse, which creates imbalance and discomfort. Many do not realize this until their improper action manifests as pain of body or soul. Today, I see my job as a healer as guiding clients on a path of self-discovery, the process of which sometimes requires provoking and digging into spiritual *ashi* points. I wonder if financial success directly relates to the level of my own awareness: Can I be fifty percent enlightened, yet receive one-hundred percent payment?

Upon graduation almost two years ago, I was offered a position by the founder of my school that made me think long and hard. Taking it would have meant a lifetime of security and an unparalleled chance to deepen my knowledge of the field; this was no ordinary job where I would be financially compensated for my time and effort. However, the opportunity came with a price I was not ready to pay. It required full dedication, to the point of sacrificing my personal life. It was the classic guru-disciple relationship, and one I was not ready to assume.

Instead I left to spend six months in South America with the woman who would later become my wife, and with the intention of meeting shamans. I imagine anyone who dedicates years to studying Oriental medicine must be attracted to things not entirely founded in logic. I once read a book written by some young Mexican doctors who had traveled to a remote area to help the indigenous population. At first they were not well received and their treatment methods were not trusted. But one doctor had studied acupuncture and began talking to the locals in the language of Oriental medicine, using the concept of "evil qi." They immediately became receptive, and not only accepted treatment, but were willing to share their own knowledge.

What I discovered in the Amazon though was quite different. Maybe it is because the jungle is so dense, so powerful, and the climate bi-seasonal, but our yin-yang and five-phase theories seemed to have little place. The shamans I met were disciplined and knowledgeable about plant spirits. But their primary job had more to do with conflict resolution, such as the use of clairvoyance to locate a thief or partner in adultery. Thus they were more feared than respected. I wonder what role the Daoist masters played in the dynastic courts of ancient China. I also wonder if the roles of real-life Amazon shamans or ancient Daoist masters are in the same galaxy of what all those hippies and new-age people define as "spiritual." In any case, my wife's family issues soon forced us to return to her hometown in Germany. It was certainly not my first choice of place to live, and my newly acquired needle qualification was not valid there. But the universe has its own design and I can do nothing but trust. We had a space available, so together we opened a healing center.

In Germany, acupuncture falls under the domain of medical doctors and naturopaths. They are not required to take any theoretical courses. Acupuncture is studied and accepted as a complimentary therapy to and within the Western framework.

My wife and I practice as "wellness practitioners." There is no clear definition as to what this implies, but it is something decidedly not medical. We are not to make diagnoses or claim to offer any medical benefits. We are not to use any instrument considered medical, but are allowed to touch the external surface of the body with our hands. We are not to prescribe any medication.

113

The long and the short is that I cannot use needles. Fortunately, there is so much more to Oriental medicine than needling. It is almost too limiting to call myself an acupuncturist. I heard a news report about a study where a scientist measured equal results with both needles and toothpicks. Myself, I mostly use a set of tuning forks for "balancing." Though I am not personally one-hundred percent sure about this method, some of my "energetically sensitive" friends swear by it. Going subtler still, I sometimes use flower essences on acupuncture points. All this is legal since there is no puncturing of the skin.

In terms of diagnostic language, we are no threat to the medical establishment. We use no measuring instruments and give no numerical data. What we do offer is insight based on the observation of nature, which is more philosophy than medicine. When I have the chance, I offer clients my five cents. Most of it flies over their head, as it did when I was on their side, but some of it seems to somehow make sense and maybe I seem impressive, as if I know something.

I started out as a massage therapist, so touch being the point of contact with clients is natural. To me, massage seems more feminine, with acupuncture being more masculine. Massage is more about listening than telling, and it can be more effective than needles in certain cases. I have studied many hands-on techniques over the years, but mostly I work intuitively. That is to say, I do not follow any set protocol but allow myself to be guided by nature.

Herbs are the most interesting part of our medicine to me, but also the biggest challenge. I eventually decided against stocking Chinese herbs, either loose or manufactured. The biggest reason was my own lack of intimacy with plants. I grew up in cities and have never experienced nature in full cycle. The shamans of the Amazon told me about difficult rites of passage they call dieta, where they eat a limited amount and stay in isolation for a number of days, focusing on one plant. If successful, the spirit of the plant communicates with the shaman, giving him the secret or information he seeks. I have seen Western people doing these dieta, but I do not believe the spirits talk to them as much. People in the jungle are wired differently, they see and feel different things.

I had one such shaman guide me in the jungle for three days. We walked for hours, and he identified more than fifty medicinal trees and plants, explaining what conditions they treated and how to administer them. For certain plants, only one specimen could be found per square mile. My not speaking the language and the jungle being so awesome, I could not take notes. (What would be the use? I could never find those plants again.) At the end of the trip I showed him my photos on my laptop, but he said he could not see the trees! In a way, this reminded me of learning Chinese herbs. I could recognize the medicinals in pictures or dried and sliced in the pharmacy, but I had never seen the whole plants or experienced the climates they grow in, let alone understood how different plants relate to each other in the wild. So instead, I offer foot-baths and herbal compresses during massages. I use food-grade herbs and they smell delicious. The result is immediate, and there are no worries about compliance or herb-med interactions.

I was the worst qi gong practitioner in school. I felt absolutely no qi moving in me when I performed the movements being taught. Once I received a treatment from a female Japanese medical qi gong practitioner that was an experience to remember: with a flick of her wrist she nailed me to the floor for six hours. There was intense pain and flash-back memories of all my previous injuries. The pain came from her qi pushing through my blockages. Amazing as it was, the experience was impersonal and ultimately I decided it was not a positive one.

I feel there is a better way to use qi, in what is called vibrational medicine. The term is vague, and you can find many websites calling it new-age hocus pocus. But these days, everyone knows a little bit about quantum physics and is aware that everything in the universe is mere vibration. Some years ago a book on water crystals made a big splash. It helped vibrational medicine by showing how thought or intention can affect form; I am most interested in this area because I feel it begins to work with the root cause of suffering.

My biggest challenge in Germany so far has been much less esoteric: language. I have to rely on my wife to translate. She is a shiatsu practitioner, a skilled communicator and understands the fundamentals of Oriental medical concepts. But still, I feel handicapped and insecure that people are not able to trust my skills.

Naturally, my ignorance of the local culture is a major hindrance to mutual trust. While yin-yang and five-phase theory may be applicable and understandable everywhere, having no knowledge about the German diet makes it challenging to give guidance on how to change eating habits. It doesn't help that I do not drink beer (I enjoy Oktoberfest; not to drink beer, but to see buxom blondes in traditional costumes!), or eat processed foods such as sausage. My wife's gluten allergy keeps bread out of the house, which leaves me just potatoes and sauerkraut. I do not follow soccer or any other ball games. We have no television in our house and our house meister think we are freaks. Maybe I am. I have not watched TV since I left New York more than fifteen years ago. My point is that I can't even make small talk to break the ice.

It maybe a stereotype, but I have found Germans to be logical, pragmatic and methodical in their approach to problems; a curious exception being homeopathy, which is widely available and accepted. There is a well-established health care system that people have to pay a significant portion of their income into, so they naturally seek out services that are covered by the system. Alternative care is something they must pay for out of their own pocket, unlike the United States where many uninsured people opt for complementary medicine because allopathic services are out of reach.

Germany is very much a Christian nation and the population is divided between those who are devoted to the church and obey doctrine without question, and those who have walked away due to their belief that the established church abuses power in the name of God. I have observed that those with this background hold a certain suspicion toward foreign spiritual traditions.

One middle-aged client, for instance, arrived with an interest in acupuncture. She said her daughter-in-law used acupuncture in her dental practice, and had recommended she try it for her migraines. She revealed that she knew the cause of her headaches (an abusive husband) and had chosen not to go to therapy because she knows what will be suggested (divorce). This, she said, is not an acceptable solution in the eyes of her church. All I could say was that I honored her decision. I did my best with a tuning fork session and gave her a bottle of essential oils for her migraines. She returned a week later saying the headaches were gone. She had one more session and a refill of the oils. She then told me that her coming to our healing center was a secret from her husband, who had asked about the different smells in the house, and also from her fellow church members, because she fears persecution for doing something they would see as bogus.

Originally, Oriental medicine was mostly a folk medicine – local healers using local herbs. The Chinese government attempted to ban the practice of it when Western medicine was introduced in the late nineteenth and early twentieth centuries, but this was generally ignored due to lack of qualified doctors in rural areas. What is now called traditional Chinese medicine is a product of Communist China, a system that does not give due credit to Daoist spirituality. A similar path was also seen in Japan, and there was a time when practitioners faced persecution.

Today, the medicines of the West and East are coming together, and the integration will advance both schools of thought. I believe that through this, acupuncture will become more universally credible. If I were more scientifically minded, and more interested in treating symptoms, I would likely feel a need to study further. But I realize my interest concerns the heart level of wellness. I am most comfortable with the Buddhist concept of karma – cause, effect, reincarnation. I believe one's salvation is dependent on having awareness of one's actions. Oriental medical concepts are a form of intelligence that help bring about peace through knowing the center. Everyone dies sooner or later. Hardship is a given, but suffering is optional.

Rather than a doctor trying to fix something, I see myself as an artist trying to guide my client to light. I want to understand, and help my client understand, the cause of their suffering. Instead of health defined as lack of disease, I want to offer the possibility of happiness despite suffering.

I recently met a truly enlightened man. He seemed a pure manifestation of love, a truly ego-less being. There was not a hint of judgment in his words or actions. When tears came in his presence, they were not from sorrow but from reconciliation. He said, "Do you know why you see darkness? Because there is so much light in the world!" So, despite the difficulty I am facing in the running of our clinic, I must be optimistic. Everyone who comes responds positively to the space we hold. There is a lot for me to learn here. I have no choice.

There is a story of an archer: A student asks how he can become a master archer. The teacher tells him to practice diligently until he has shot 100,000 bull's eyes. Many years pass and the student finally reaches the goal. He tells his teacher he has completed the task. The master tells him he now must shoot the bull's eye 100,000 times without using a bow and arrow.

You work because the work calls you, but in the end the only act is no action, letting go. I've heard the Chinese call it *wu wei*.

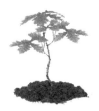

FORMATIVE EXPERIENCES
BY EMILY SMITH

I have had an acupuncture license for nearly twenty years. So why am I writing a chapter for a book on "green" acupuncturists? Well, read on to find out.

I graduated from the American College of Traditional Chinese Medicine in San Francisco, California, in October 1992 with a degree in acupuncture and herbology. I studied Chinese acupuncture and I enjoyed the strong stimulation of the thick needles. I spent a lot of time needling myself to learn which points and techniques caused specific results or sensations.

However, I noticed that I could not really control the amount of stimulation. Some of my patients were happy with the strong "*hibiki*" or *de qi* feeling, while others were distinctly disturbed by it. In my third year of school, I started to learn about Japanese needles, guide tubes and the importance of palpating before, during and after treatment. Palpation became my primary focus and continues to reliably give me valuable information during treatments. Developing manual dexterity has been an ongoing process and I cannot emphasize how important it is to assess a whole-body picture.

The day after graduation in 1992, I hopped on a plane for Japan. I had found a national hospital in Tsukuba, Ibaraki Prefecture, with an intern program; never mind that I knew hardly any Japanese. For the next four months, my time was divided between two clinics and culture shock.

The first clinic was the beautiful state-of-the-art Tsukuba College of Technology. It is actually an acupuncture clinic, but they knew better than to say that outright. In Japan, acupuncture and moxibustion are only beginning to return to the status they deserve. Well before World War II, Western medicine became the respected norm, and acupuncture and moxibustion were looked down on as folk medicine. The hospital I interned at was the first of its kind in the country. Doctors and acupuncturists worked side-by-side, first giving a biomedical diagnosis and then recommending acupuncture.

National health insurance in Japan will pay for acupuncture for only six symptoms: back pain, arthritis, neck and shoulder syndrome, whiplash, knee pain, and nerve pain. For most Japanese practitioners, a referral from a doctor is rather unprofitable, so many combine acupuncture with a Japanese form of chiropractic that is more readily accepted by national health insurance. When I arrived, the lack of acceptance and popularity of acupuncture was quite a surprise, to say the least. In any case, the facility at the college was beautiful, but for my purposes the treatments were too biomedical in their approach.

My second internship was at an aging hole-in-the-wall in Shinjuku, Tokyo. I had heard stories about traditional Japanese medicine practiced in places like this, where treatment extends beyond the body to patients' lives; where the practitioner notices how the patients fold their clothes and leave their slippers, how they get up from the table after treatment, how they greet the practitioner and the clinic staff, whether they are habitually late, and as their condition improves, how they put more energy and attention into themselves, their surroundings, and their relationships. This cramped clinic brought that image to life!

Even though I could not understand the words spoken, I could feel the energy and this was enough to keep me intrigued. The practitioner, Togasaki-sensei, used silver and gold needles, sharpened by hand and sterilized by autoclave after each use. Sharpening needles is hard work that takes time and concentration, so a big part of the interns' job was, and still is, sharpening needles. Skip ahead to 2010 and Togasaki-sensei is still using his original method but has begun to integrate thicker, sometimes stainless steel needles, saying results come quicker. Occasionally patients ask for disposable needles, so there are always some kept on hand.

The Shinjuku clinic also taught tai ji quan, and the acupuncturists, assistants and many patients regularly attended classes. I was immediately put off by the soft, fluid style of tai ji they taught, but soon realized my hard and forceful nature (and treatment style) could definitely benefit from some gentleness. This practice, I like to think, has helped me connect my breath, movements and mind; it is like a moving meditation. Initially, the forms felt robotic, but gradually, over the years,

119

they became so natural that wavering from the flow felt awkward and unnatural. Partner exercises were also taught to help us focus on our own levels of relaxation or tension, and to help us feel these aspects in another, be it opponent, partner or patient. Only by relaxing yourself can you perceive where someone else is stuck and forcing - the root of all discomfort. The teacher had us check our tension levels in specific areas, like wrists, elbows, hips or knees. Only by understanding my own tight, blind or numb spots can I begin to understand how to focus my intention and feel someone else's areas of tension or relaxation.

In between tai ji classes, I observed treatments at the clinic. The main practitioner spoke no English, so I mostly just watched like a hawk and tried my best to understand his style. The language barrier was far more difficult than I had anticipated, but I did learn a lot about how to organize and run an efficient and economical clinic. Now, almost twenty years later, Togasaki-sensei's style has evolved significantly and he has clearly settled on a specific approach to treatment. Being able to see this process has fundamentally influenced my own growth.

Finally, I was swamped with culture shock. I had dreamed of traveling to Japan but actually being here was incredibly difficult. In hindsight, I can see how I suppressed parts of myself that I deemed inappropriate because I wanted to fit in. Gradually, as my Japanese improved and I made friends, I was able to be myself again. This worn-down clinic changed my life forever and I have been in Japan ever since.

Life Happens

After about a year, in February 1993, I had to return to America for the California licensing exams. Although in some ways I felt ready to start practicing, I was overwhelmingly drawn to make a serious study of Japanese language and acupuncture. I decided to live in Japan and try to make a living teaching English until I could attend acupuncture school there. Despite the crippling language barrier, the failing economy and the often infuriating cultural differences, I returned in September 1993. Although I felt I was truly following my heart, not being able to practice was aggravating. Also, the biomedical model had changed traditional Oriental medicine almost beyond recognition in Japan, so it was very difficult to find like-minded students and practitioners. The Shinjuku clinic seemed to be the only place of its kind, so I continued to intern there.

So, my life and learning took the scenic route. I had to learn how to split myself between Japan and America, and then family and work.

Marriage happened in 1994 and April Fool's Day is our anniversary, just to keep us humble. Our son Yuhta was born in August 1995 and our daughter Luna in 1998. I was a "Christmas cake," which means I was well past the age of twenty-five at marriage. Old maids who cannot manage to get married by the ripe age of twenty-five are called Christmas cake in Japan. (Get it? Twenty-four is still not too late.) This old-fashioned way of looking at things really did not have a major influence on me, but I mention it to give you an idea of the inanity I encountered here. Many modern Japanese women hold off or refuse marriage, and they laugh at the absurdity of the expression.

Marriage and kids are amazing teachers because they get you where it counts, and then, if you are willing, get you to laugh about it! My family is perfect for me, of course, but the pertinent part here is that, although I had no license to practice, I had some willing practice models; primarily my husband. He does not like needles and is terribly sensitive to massage, which only made me further develop my hands, a skill vital to my current practice. Whereas my Chinese professors in America barely touched the patient before needling, I palpate my patients' entire body before and after. I also periodically check for changes during the treatment. Thankfully, I can now rely on my hands to determine where to place needles, or can use my fingers to do the job instead, if necessary.

But back to the kids. It felt very natural to put most of my activities aside to bring the world to life for them, as my mother had done for me, but by the time my daughter was in first grade I was ready for more challenges. Attending Japanese acupuncture school had always been in the back of my mind, but I definitely did not want to leave my kids in a lurch, emotionally or physically. Eventually I decided to go, knowing I would never forgive myself, or my family, if I did not pursue my dream. Plus, we all would benefit from my new and improved training, enthusiasm for life, and improved Japanese skills.

I applied and was accepted to the school closest to Tsukuba, only ninety minutes from home, door to door. Of course this is not close at all, but many people here commute further than that each day... frogs in a pot of slowly heating water, right? From the get go, school was pure hell. I probably made it more difficult than it needed to be, but I was used to getting good grades and was totally prepared to work hard. What I was not ready for was the language difficulty. The school I attended boasts a nearly perfect passing rate for the national exam, so all the students are really pressured to be prepared. Bottom line, tests galore: nearly every day I had a quiz or test on material I had learned the previous week.

Although being able to read and write Japanese at a high-school level is sufficient for Japanese acupuncture school, my own skills were far below that. Of course, I had studied the TCM bit of acupuncture before, but memorizing all the kanji characters for the anatomy, physiology and clinical pathology, not to mention the acupoints, was a constant race against time. Even having studied, I failed tests and had to retake them. But I did pass, and actually became able to accept passing with a terrible grade. My pride and confidence took a real beating and I understood why so many Japanese students get fed up with the system - you have to memorize everything for the test but the actual exam is short and concise, covering only a small portion of what you have stuffed in your head.

What kept me going was the undying belief that I could do anything I set my mind to. I absolutely had to get that license or I would be doomed to life as a housewife! I had never attempted anything so constantly demanding and difficult – the commute, the unending demands of being a mom, the personal need to prove myself to my family, my classmates and myself. Japanese acupuncture school tested me from every angle for three years.

But in the end, I passed the national exam. Finally I had a license I could use!

In February of 2009 I received my licenses in the mail. I was set and had a plan. I started hunting for a reasonable space and organizing my lists of necessary equipment. By September my clinic, which had been a company cafeteria, was ready to go. I wanted a conspicuous location but not the high rent, so I settled on the first floor of an apartment building set back from the street. The place has a large room that I use as a yoga studio, two very spacious treatment rooms, a bathroom, office, storage room, kitchen and eight parking spaces. It was not exactly conveniently located but it was very spacious and reasonably priced. The down side is that it is off the street, so only people who know there is an office there actually come in.

So the office was ready and I was set; all I needed was patients. I had signs up, but they did not bring in much business. I spread the word to my friends and hoped they would pass it on. Slowly people started calling.

My first patient was a friend. She had been treated with acupuncture before for infertility, but was coming to me for stress-related fatigue and Meniere's syndrome. I was determined to be professional to prevent the situation from becoming too familiar, which I feared would lead to haggling over payment. She actually laughed at me in my white coat (almost all practitioners here wear the white coat), saying it felt like we were playing house. Unfazed, I proceeded with the treatment. She was impressed with the painless needling, saying it helped her neck and shoulder tension. We agreed on a reasonable, but reduced rate. I really just wanted people to keep coming back, so I was willing to compromise on the fee. After 1½ years, my business is almost completely word-of-mouth, so it pays to keep people talking positively about me. Tsukuba is small and I have been here long enough to have lots of friends who refer people to me.

Plans and Reality

When I opened my doors I had this great idea, I thought, "I'll treat people, not conditions." We are energetic creatures, influenced by a constant stream of stimuli, including people, beliefs, habits and memories. People and their bodies change all day, every day, and I want to treat the whole person on as many levels as I am capable of. The idea of a fixed menu, with a specific time limit and an accompanying price, seems to put the emphasis on time and money rather than on delivering effective medicine.

But the reality has been that people come with a specific complaint and want some immediate relief. Initially I tried to use my whole-body method on everybody, naively thinking that the symptom would resolve itself along the way. The person who really made this misconception clear to me wanted to be treated for chronic stiff shoulders. This very healthy and otherwise vibrant 53-year-old woman was a concert pianist. She had been visiting the local chiropractor because of the strong massage that preceded the treatment. This massage effectively, albeit temporarily, relieved her shoulder stiffness. I saw the stiffness as a deficiency of yin with yang rising.

The treatment was going fine until the November cold began to seep into my new treatment room. I had a ceiling heater and a hot pad for her feet but the floor was cold. Soon her extremities were chilled and nothing I did seemed to improve her imbalance. The treatment went on too long and she left repeating her initial mantra – that her condition was unique and difficult to treat. My whole-body method

123

had not allowed me to focus enough on her main complaint to gain her faith.

I have since perfected my heating system to make sure the elements are not a limiting factor. And now, especially when patients are new, I include some muscle tests to clarify for the patient and myself as accurately as possible where the stiffness, tension and weaknesses are located. I also try to get an idea of how much energy they are putting into their condition. Set attitudes, resistance to change, fear of relaxing and lifestyle comfort zones allow symptoms to linger. The pianist's repeated insistence that her case was difficult should have set off sirens about resistance to feeling better.

Gradually, I am learning how combine whole body treatments with quick and effective symptomatic relief.

Beliefs Matter

I have discovered that people develop symptoms for very good reasons! Discomfort can often be a coping mechanism for work-related stress and fatigue, poor posture, diet and lifestyle patterns, relationship difficulty or fading dreams. In my short experience I have seen people, once they start to show improvement, create some resistance, often emotional or even unconscious, to feeling better. Especially with long-standing conditions, which are so well woven into people's lives, freedom from the symptom means reweaving a big part of their routine and relationships. Migraines, weight-loss and Meniere's syndrome are a few of the issues I have seen resist recovery.

One patient with Meniere's syndrome came in complaining of terrible vertigo nearly every day. Her symptoms were not new and the medication she had been taking has not been effective. When I first examined her, I noticed numerous open and half-healed sores on her legs, arms and abdomen. I initially suspected chronic inflammation due to compromised circulation, as in diabetes, but she said they were flea bites! Her cat was infested but since she did not want to use flea powder, the whole family suffered. What I really wanted to ask was, "What about the stress caused by these constant sores?"

The first treatment was too strong and she said she was overwhelmed by the release of energy. The second treatment she reported as very satisfying and left feeling much better. She had begun to talk about the stress in her life and how being busy made her head spin. Menstrual difficulties also contributed to her symptoms but she could not pinpoint anything she might be doing to exacerbate her condition.

Unfortunately, the third treatment was delayed because of a long winter holiday. She came in exhausted, worried about her two children who do not like to be alone with their elderly grandmother, her mother-in-law who lived with them, and complained about mornings being too hectic. I suggested that getting up just fifteen minutes before the family does might give her some much needed personal time, but she said she would rather get the extra sleep.

She relaxed into the treatment but soon I realized the classical music I was playing was too frenetic. I changed it but it was too late, she said the room was spinning. I did a gentle grounding technique and asked her to rest quietly for a while, but she still left feeling somewhat dizzy. She scheduled her next appointment for after her next period, despite my suggestion that preparing her body for menstruation might make the rest of the month easier to manage.

After she left, I thought about her condition and lifestyle. It seemed she was not interested in changing, at least not in the ways I had suggested. She kept coming for a while but the seventh treatment was her last. The intervals between treatments had been so long she could not feel any lasting effect. I had suggested weekly treatments to help her start feeling consistently better but she declined, explaining the time and effort of getting to the clinic was too much for her. So I was left feeling unable to help her. I thought her condition would improve with some consistent attention, but her life situation and beliefs about her place in it could not support her efforts.

Beliefs are often limiting in their nature, and are usually reinforced through experiences, cultural paradigms and relationships. Outsmarting the beliefs and gently reprogramming fixed responses to allow for a broader comfort zone takes preparation. I try, gradually, to make it clear to myself and my patients that understanding the imbalance behind the symptom will provide clues to graceful natural change and long-lasting relief.

Not everyone can appreciate this. I had a young runner who came in only once. He had just moved to Tsukuba for a graduate program and was also a star on the track team. He had no friends yet and no real connections in the community. During his first week he tore his Achilles tendon. After surgery he found my website and wanted me to heal his tendon. He had been treated before and evidently thought one treatment would do it. When I explained he would have to come several times, he balked and never returned. I never even had the chance to suggest this type of "accident" does not happen suddenly. Gradual stiffening and the stress and anticipation of success or failure probably set him up for a tragic injury.

Western medicine has pills and surgery for relatively quick relief, but as an acupuncturist I need to draw the patient out of their dis-comfort zone and back into a, for lack of a better expression, empowered state of health. Rewriting the unexamined belief script may not be a conscious effort, but gradually, as the patient learns to regularly relax in their body, natural wellness can begin to outweigh the older patterns.

Many patients have simply lost confidence in their ability to manage their health. They are entirely focused on being fixed. I remember the first person who said she felt "betrayed" by her body. She had experienced uterine tumors, undergone surgery and was on hormone replacements that made her feel bloated, and had sent her into early menopause. Her husband had taken a job that took him away from her and her teenage children to be near his aging mother. She said she felt betrayed by her body, but did she really mean her husband? She came in for relaxation but soon admitted, shyly, that what she really wanted was ear acupuncture for weight loss. She was not interested in exercise and fretted about her habit of staying up late nibbling on chocolates while surfing the web.

Modern medicine had encouraged a mind-body split by providing treatment that removed the tumors, but left her with a very limited view of health and well-being. Her experiences with disease significantly diminished her incentive to take responsibility for her health. I had hoped my role would be to assist my patients in understanding their patterns of tension, weakness, and dis-ease, and as they regained ease and comfort, they could take the reins for themselves, making informed choices about health, treatment frequency and lifestyle changes.

This woman came regularly for quite a while, although she continued to behave as if acupuncture in her ears twice a month would fix her weight issues. Maybe I should have talked more about her attitude, helping her develop some courage to look at dietary changes and exercise as exciting possibilities, rather than an uphill battle. She discontinued treatment to enter an English teacher's training program, which had been her life-long dream. Unfortunately, while working so hard toward her goal, her body was increasingly burdened and she ended up hospitalized for exhaustion. The lesson here is that we need to make friends with our body. It can be our most trusted and loyal companion, but if ignored, it surely will create havoc.

What is acupuncture good for?

Visiting acupuncture websites, I often find lists of World Health Organization-approved symptoms that respond positively to acupuncture. These lists, although necessary to help patients decide if they want to try acupuncture, seem like a fabrication, bending Oriental medicine to fit biomedical symptoms. I was first drawn to this medicine because it seemed to side-step the symptom and teach people about patterns, about the tendencies that create imbalance, deficiency or excess. Learning how to live in our body should not be a mystery or a test. This wisdom is available freely, so from my perspective, the patient and his or her body are doing the healing.

That said, I need detailed information about where to take the treatment on a given day. Relevant questions can bring the patient into their body, but anyone who has treated knows that the descriptions patients give of how they are feeling are not always reliable. Pain and suffering cloud our perceptions and as a symptom lingers, its effects gradually narrow our thoughts and beliefs about the body.

So I use my hands, eyes, ears and intuition (okay my nose may be involved too, but I do not rely on it especially) to gather information. Palpation is the primary tool of Japanese acupuncture and I use it constantly, from initially taking the pulse to palpating the whole body before doing anything else. The patient may say their left shoulder is really tense but my palpation could reveal significant tension in the right as well. Most patients arrive with an idea about their condition and want to talk about it. Initially, I ask about sensations or symptoms, and these specific questions help me either confirm my suspicions or aid me in developing my senses. After I get to know the person, I need to ask less and can rely on my perceptions more.

Patients who are willing to talk about their symptoms in detail can be a mixed blessing. I know one woman who will talk endlessly about her sons' troubles but never get to her own. So I try to suggest that her preoccupation with her son is an obstacle to both her and her son's development or recovery. Then there is the over-worked dad who can hardly bring himself to mention a problem beyond the obligatory "stiff shoulders." Even after a very successful treatment (from my perspective successful means the tension I felt initially is replaced by a certain amount of release and a change in breathing depth and rhythm.), he rarely offers any comment. Completely annoyed with this patient, I conferred with a colleague who suggested he might just have low sensitivity and suggested I use stronger stimulation. This was great advice. I had been using the thinnest Japanese needles on everyone because I did not want to cause any jolts, so I had never even considered stronger stimulation. But the reality is that some patients need to feel something specific to understand their body's reaction or lack thereof. After nearly two years, I am still using Japanese needles, but now use ones that are thick enough to hold a moxa ball on the handle and can produce good *de qi*.

I want to keep developing so I can efficiently assess patients' patterns of disharmony by relying as little as possible on verbal information.

Having a Clinic

Living in Japan has meant a very cozy but cluttered living environment. Most people who have never visited the country have no idea how small and cramped most Japanese homes are. In contrast, my clinic is spacious, uncluttered and very refreshing. After nearly twenty years of waiting, I wanted to have everything perfect, so right off the bat I cleaned and prepared my clinic every morning. Even if I had no patients scheduled, I wanted to be ready. Prepare for the unexpected. This work reassures me that I can relax and focus 100 percent on the patient, rather than searching for the items I need. I work alone, so it will be me who has to dash out for the extra moxa sticks or box of tissues.

Perhaps I will change, but at this point my mental and physical condition is very important. I get plenty of sleep, good food and rejuvenating stimulation in the form of yoga, meditation, time with my kids and friends, and ongoing internships and studies.

The idea of treating patients with acupuncture all day, every day has never appealed to me. For the most part I just treat one patient at a time. The Japanese practitioners I am familiar with, on the other hand, cram four or five beds into a small room, separate everyone with curtains, and move people in and out every half hour. My teacher treats this way but he has three assistants. There are also practitioners who boast nine years of continuous practice, with no days off and no vacations! My patient load is quite light in comparison but I am happy with my results so far.

I have also opened a yoga studio. Yoga seemed useful for a few reasons. It is good for people who already feel pretty decent or for those who do not want acupuncture, and it is good for me too. Like tai ji, yoga is a great way to get out of one's head and into ones body. Yoga is humbling, challenging and gets most people moving in ways they had forgotten are possible. I had been practicing for twenty years and had never thought about teaching, but when a nearly perfect space presented itself, I jumped at the opportunity. My classes continue to grow and the low prices surprise many people. My first yoga teacher had really low prices. Her idea was if the cost was affordable, students can come a lot, get better fast and feel good sooner. I like this and want students to value the practice more than they worry about the cost.

I thought there would be more overlap between acupuncture patients and yoga students, but what has happened is that people who want a whole-body treatment come several times a week to yoga class, and people who have a specific symptom or condition come for acupuncture. Traditional texts suggest that acupuncture, moxibustion, herbs, massage and lifestyle guidance can be used even in the absence of outright disease. If we expect our bodies to stay healthy and vital into old age, it makes sense to have a knowledgeable teacher whose guidance we trust. I am happy to provide this for people and I try to encourage them to start with acupuncture or massage instead of forcing themselves into yoga. Gradually, my yoga students have started asking questions about certain conditions and some have come for acupuncture.

Speed Bumps

Speed bumps are conspicuous obstructions in the road that are intended to catch a traveler's attention and slow him or her down. If you go too fast over them, they really hit hard. If, on the other hand, you travel at a reasonable pace, the bumps are simply safety reminders and are not major obstacles. In my first year, I was driving too fast. I was eager and excited, and although I thought a lot, I encountered many unexpected speed bumps.

I will never forget the first time I lost a phone call. A man called, seemed interested, we talked and he hung up. I did not get his phone number, suggest a convenient time or do anything else to encourage him to come in. Now I know to ask about a caller's condition, try to schedule an appointment or at least get contact information. Since then, I have not lost another call.

But a bump I keep running into has been getting patients to reschedule. My teacher in Tokyo always tells the patient when to come back. Some people are twice a week, others once every three weeks. He has nearly thirty years experience and authority behind him. Some famous practitioners here see patients with serious conditions twice a day,

129

every day, until they feel better. This kind of treatment frequency is a luxury I would love to suggest but I do not, yet. Some people happily reschedule, others prefer to call when they are ready. Occasionally, someone goes too long and comes back in really bad shape. Then I explain that regular treatments help the body remember a healthy state.

A Japanese expression says that when you open a new clinic, you eat cold rice for three years, meaning that it takes about three years before you will start seeing a profit.

I checked the other clinics in the area and set my prices at the same level. The going rate is, drum roll please, 4,000 yen (about $45) and my treatments take about an hour and fifteen minutes. My initial priority was to get people in the door rather than make a fortune, but because I spend more time with each patient than most local practitioners, I do look forward to the time when I can reasonably raise my rates. I have heard of acupuncturists here who treat by time or symptom, such as in ten or fifteen minute intervals, or charge a certain amount for back pain and a different amount for a stomach ache. Most of these acupuncturists use a fixed protocol to get patients in and out the door quickly.

But most of my clients are new to acupuncture, and are not thrilled to be paying for something above and beyond their mandatory health insurance. So, I am optimistic that the popularity of acupuncture in Japan will grow, as it has in the rest of the world, and that building patient confidence and loyalty will eventually pay dividends for the profession as a whole.

I thought long and hard about the name for my clinic, since after nearly twenty years of waiting I wanted it to be really great. Unfortunately, the muse of great business names did not visit me and I chose a loser name. Most Japanese acupuncturists until recently just used their last name, like Ishihara Acupuncture. But I wanted something inspiring and creative, so I ran ideas past many friends and my family before deciding on Holistic Health Tsukuba. Almost immediately upon deciding, my daughter astutely renamed it Holy Hell. Holistic is not a familiar English word here so I have to explain it, and it is just too long in general. I am now brainstorming again.

Simply opening my doors was a huge success for me. It got me out of the mother-housewife rut that was threatening my sanity. For all the time and anticipation I put into this endeavor, it seems to be unfolding perfectly. Of course there is a learning curve but the satisfaction I get from the process is more than I could have hoped for.

It has always made sense that we should listen to our bodies and learn how to find balance in all areas of our lives; now that longevity and wellness are becoming more valued by the mainstream, maybe it will be easier for more of us to enjoy vibrant health into old age.

The physiological effects of this shift in values may be years away, but gradually the seeds of change are germinating. Scientific evidence that suggests that acupuncture is effective may reassure many people, but I am betting that most cannot wait that long. Why wait for the cancer to show up on the CT scan when you can live a healthy, comfortable life without fear of any degenerative diseases? That is what health can and should be, assisting and trusting our body and its natural resources. Making sensible lifestyle choices seems to be the best way to give ourselves ongoing wellness. Twenty years ago when I started this adventure, some part of me knew the path would take me where I needed to go: toward empowering myself and my patients to manage their health.

Disease does not happen to us, we either create it or eliminate it with our thoughts, lifestyle and activities, and the key to a high-energy lifestyle is simply learning to tap the energy we have bundled up in patterns of stress and strain. Maintaining energy levels is all about balance. It is natural to be up some of the time and to wind down at other times. The trouble is that there are some times when it is more convenient to be up or down than others. Most of us have gradually learned to ignore or override the messages our body and mind send to each other. Relearning how to tune into these signals takes time and patience, but the dividends will sustain us into old age. Understanding the way our body and mind work, and how they are affected by certain stressors, such as food, the environment or even people, can free up enough energy to help us effectively choose the times we are up or down. By maintaining a good balance between the two, we will never reach the stage of complete exhaustion that leads to serious illness.

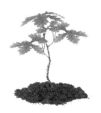

FINDING A VOICE
BY CARL STIMSON

Humans have a tendency to focus on their weaknesses and ignore their strengths. Struggle pushes us to learn, while competency can lead to complacency. Who is more likely to be an expert on all the different ways to stay in shape, the person whose metabolism keeps them naturally thin or the soul who cannot seem to keep pounds off? Who is more likely to explore the galaxy of spiritualities, one who is content with life or the person who is constantly flailing for equilibrium? The solutions we settle on might be off-base or lead to their own difficulties, but the desire to learn, to overcome, springs from deficiency and doubt.

I discovered early on in my Chinese medicine career that one of the natural talents I was not blessed with was the ability to attract patients. I remember feeling hurt and confused when I watched classmates work through full schedules in the intern clinic while I sat idle, fretting that I would not make my quota for the semester.

Before we started treating the public in the intern clinic in the fourth semester, I felt very comfortable at school. The curriculum was challenging but I quickly realized I could handle the intellectual aspect of Chinese medicine, and was actually quite good at it. Members of my family going back several generations have had academic degrees, and at home my parents made it clear they knew I could do well in school and expected good marks. So with both nature and nurture on my side, I never had much trouble with formal learning. In my first couple of semesters I rode this easy wave, soaking up information and sniffing around the subtle logic of the Chinese system. Doing well in class felt good, but in my heart I knew accomplishments in this sphere came without much effort on my part.

This complacency is probably why my struggles to attract patients, both before and after graduation, came as such a shock. For a while I wallowed in bitterness and self-pity, feeling my success in the classroom should have automatically led to patients beating down my door. I do not think I was ever silly enough to think this consciously, but in retrospect that is what was going on under the surface.

Eventually, slowly, I accepted the reality of the situation. And with that I became able to begin the search for answers. I looked both internally to try to discover what was preventing me from connecting with patients, and externally to examine what successful practitioners were doing. I could see how some of my personality traits were keeping me from attracting patients, but looking outside for role models was confusing at first. Now, however, I have a few ideas on why patients flock to certain practitioners.

First, myself. Despite an inner life so active it sometimes feels like I am burning up (Scorpio, Snake), most people tell me I come across as calm and relaxed. Although I hid behind shyness as a child, this outer quiet is not a false face. There is simply something in my personality that prefers to hang back and observe, to make connections slowly – no matter what is blazing inside. Although this modus operandi has worked well enough for me in the slow, careful dance of forming personal relationships, it has proved a handicap in making bonds with patients, which must usually be done in the first treatment if you want to see them again.

Things that for my whole life I considered positive parts of my personality were now having terrible effects. For instance, I had always prided myself on my ability to treat people with respect and goodwill. But with my reserved personality, this often manifested as a live-and-let-live attitude; if someone was not interested in seeing or doing things my way, I could easily accept it and let them go on as they pleased. This easy-going style, when placed in the clinic, was a disaster. My follow-up with patients was weak and my treatment plans lacked conviction. Patients floated in, I treated them once and they floated away, never to be seen again. Not angry, not unsatisfied, but definitely not hooked.

I was not completely hopeless. Like all practitioners, I had patients who inexplicably loved me and credited me with doing great things for them. And I had normal ones who came in with a problem and I helped them deal with it over a series of treatments. But I knew I was losing too many patients.

During my first year of practice I lived in Boston. Fittingly for me, I went against the stream by living in the city and working in the suburbs. It was autumn of 2008 when I finally got my license and was ready to practice. Just months before, my wife and I had moved back to the United States after a year in China, and on the Fourth of July in Butte, Montana, we shook Barack Obama's hand at a campaign stop. My wife declared this an excellent omen for our new life in the States.

As the year grew colder however, the U.S. economy tanked, the stock market plunged, unemployment soared and my hopes for a successful career shriveled, though I was too scared to admit this to myself at the time. During these frustrating and hopeless months, one of the few bright spots was that I had the good fortune to work under three very successful practitioners. Two were my bosses at clinics I worked at and one was a well-known acupuncturist I interned under. Being around them and seeing how they interacted with patients helped me learn some basic characteristics of what leads to a successful practice.

Before I get into that though, I would like to clear up any possible misunderstanding of my motivations. This desire to attract and keep patients was not simply lust for name and gain, nor did it spring purely from a deep-seated hope to help as many people as possible. It was both of these, and there were other things behind it as well: anxiety about being able to support a family, curiosity to explore and learn by experience, desire to increase the acceptance of our medicine, and simply an enjoyment of building relationships with patients and wanting to do more of it. My motivations, in other words, were muddy.

But back to these three mentors and what they taught me. I am going to link each one with teaching me one important aspect of building solid working relationships with patients. In reality, this is too simple, as all of them were skillful in dealing with patients in many ways. For the sake of this essay, however, I am going to break things down in this way.

My first boss, Robert, was an inspiration close to my heart. He was just a few years older than me, and had been practicing for just about two years when he and his business partner hired me. In that short time, they had built a thriving community acupuncture clinic that saw close to forty patients per day between them. I was hired because they were looking to expand their hours to evenings and weekends. Wow, I thought during the interviews, this is exactly the place I want to work.

They are providing affordable care to heaps of people and they are making a solid living.

I ended up taking on only two shifts at this clinic (in retrospect, a mistake) and the start of my evening hours overlapped with the end of Robert's daytime shift. He showed a lot of concern with getting me up and running, and would set aside plenty of time to talk about how things were going and offer advice.

Robert strongly emphasized the need for clearly communicating with patients, especially when they first came in. Thinking about it now, laying out a clear treatment plan during the first visit and giving people an idea of the progress they should expect seems like a no-brainer, but it was not something anyone had ever sat down and explained to me; not in practice management classes nor at the intern clinic.

However, Robert took things a step further and emphasized that patients had to be "sold" the treatment plan. At first I was put off by this seemingly greed-based attitude, but I eventually came to agree wholeheartedly that salesmanship is exactly what is needed with new patients. Now wait – I can picture some of you curling your lip in distaste – let me explain. As I see it now, selling a product is neither a good or a bad thing. It can, of course, be harmful, such as the proverbial used car salesman foisting a lemon off on an ignorant buyer. However, a dictionary defines "sell" as, "The exchange of... services for an amount of money," with no mention of greed or trickery.

For a patient, the decision to get acupuncture is in part an economic one involving time and money. If a person believes the benefit they will gain from acupuncture is significantly less than what they must give away to get it, they will not schedule appointments. But since most people have very little knowledge of acupuncture, there is a great danger that this decision will be made in at least partial ignorance. Therefore, it is a practitioner's duty to explain fully what patients will have to do as their part of the bargain and the benefits they are likely to gain by doing so. If we fail in this, they may decide mistakenly that acupuncture cannot help them, which would be akin to negligence on our part. People come to us looking for help. If we believe we can provide this and do not try our best to convince them that acupuncture provides an opportunity to heal, is this any less of a mistake than needling SP-6 in a pregnant woman or giving ginseng to a guy with excess heat?

So I started putting Robert's advice into practice. I tried to tell patients as clearly as I could my thoughts on how much I could help and how long it would take. And I made progress. I could see in patients' eyes that they had a grasp of the choice they were faced with. Not everyone chose to take the treatment plan I laid out, but those who did, I felt more secure with, and less like every appointment was some kind of win-or-lose showdown. But still I felt something was missing. I doubted success depended fully on such a clear cut and logical solution. There must be another element, something more intangible.

The second clinic I worked at during my first year of practice did mostly massage and I was the only acupuncturist. My boss, Frank, was an incredible bodyworker. He had skill, no doubt, but the thing that amazed me about him was his ability to see people. Everybody who studies a healing art gradually internalizes the system they practice so minor clues – how someone stands or the way a person laughs – provide deep insight into the body and mind. But I have met a few people in my short career who seem to have x-ray vision. Their powers of observation go beyond training and familiarity; it is something inborn, I believe. Frank had this ability.

I loved to watch how Frank made use of his talents; it never ceased to fascinate me. Soon after meeting new patients, with very little talking or palpation, he would be able to tell them profound things about their bodies, minds, health issues, bad habits and positive attributes. And not only could he point out what was going on with someone, Frank had the ability to show people what a new-and-improved state would feel like, if only in a small way. With just a few nudges to adjust a person's posture and a couple words to suggest what kind of changes these adjustments would bring, he had people he had met just ten minutes before seeing that sweeping changes were possible. They were, in a word, inspired. Heck, I was inspired and I was just watching from the corner.

Frank was always on me about treatment plans as well, but I knew his success did not come from simply laying out clearly how often a person would have to return. His patients were hooked by what he was able to tell them about themselves. When Frank worked on me or other staff members, I was able to follow his train of thought better, since I was more intimately acquainted with the subjects, but even still, the leaps he made and their accuracy always left me shaking my head.

136

The inspiration Frank provided was not amazing because he was revealing mysterious secrets, but because he told people things they had always known about themselves but had lain just under the surface, unable to be expressed. "Through a glass, darkly," as the Bible says.

Clear communication about treatment plans and expectations gives patients the freedom to make an informed choice, it is a cerebral, rational avenue. Frank's method, on the other hand, offered people something more fundamental: hope. And showing people what was possible led to faith, which kept them coming back to see him not for months, but for years.

"But wait!" you say, "What am I supposed to do? I don't have x-ray vision." Neither do I, and unfortunately this is where things get less clear cut. Finding the thing inside oneself that can kindle hope in others is not easy. Frank found it in a special skill set, others may have different talents that fill this role, an ability to inspire with words or merely a presence that bring patients some peace and allows them to see through their current fog.

As for me, I am still searching. I know people are soothed by my calm exterior, and patients have told me it has helped them stay steady amidst the ups and downs of the healing process. But this is a slow-burning gift and it usually takes a while for people to recognize it. Probably my gifts require a larger time investment to allow for proper ripening. I am learning to accept this – but my fiery inner self still craves something a little flashier.

The treatment plans Robert taught me to value addressed the mind and the inspiration I saw Frank wield made the heart bloom, but what about the gut, the base, the foundation?

My third lesson about successful interactions with patients came from interning under an established acupuncturist during my first year of practice. Kiiko is incredibly talented with the needle, there can be no doubt, but the biggest lesson I took away from my time with her was the value of determination, of not giving up.

Before observing Kiiko work, my idea of an acupuncture treatment went like this: greet the patient, go through the four examinations, decide on what methods to use, give the treatment, book the next appointment and say goodbye. If the patient felt better after the treatment, great. If not, one could needle a few more local points or put some ear seeds in, but the best thing to do was encourage the patient to come back as soon as possible, since acupuncture treatments build on each other. After my experience in Kiiko's clinic, settling for this seems at best lazy and at worst negligent.

If I were to describe Kiiko's treatment style in one word, I think I would choose "aggressive." Usually this word, when associated with acupuncture, conjures up images of painful needle stimulation and heavy amounts of direct moxibustion, but this is not what I mean. When presented with a complaint or when a painful reflex was found by palpation, she would try to eliminate it with a persistence that was almost thrilling to watch.

Relief of seventy to one-hundred percent by the time the patient left the clinic was optimal, improvement of around fifty percent was grudgingly acceptable, and anything less than thirty percent elicited fervent apologies and near begging to allow her to try again in a follow-up treatment. Kiiko's treatments came in multiple stages: she needled patients lying on their back, front, one or both sides and sometimes sitting up. The improvement rates mentioned above were for the end of the treatment, but even in the initial part, before the patient was left to rest lying supine with needles in, she would shoot for forty to fifty percent improvement.

Does pressing this point help? *A little.* What about this one? *Better.* If I add this point over here? *Better still.* All right, needles in – how is it now? *Not bad.* Stimulate – what about now? *Not much different.* Change the angle and stimulate again – any improvement? *Oh, that's quite a bit better.* Good, Carl moxa these two points and follow me to the next patient.

There were times when it dragged on. A stiff shoulder was fifty percent looser after an hour-long treatment but she wanted more. Point after point, moxa cone after moxa cone, looking for a little more relief. Even the patient was ready to go, telling Kiiko that he was doing good and would come back next week. As I stood there and watched, I knew I would have let things be long before, that I would have been happy with a thirty percent improvement. But Kiiko drove on and in the end she usually got what she wanted. Most patients left feeling at least seventy-five percent better, often shaking their heads in amazement while they handed over their payment and booked their next appointment.

In part, Kiiko's ability to keep chipping away at pain and tender reflexes is due to the techniques she uses. They allow for an incredible amount of flexibility and here-and-now practicality compared to standard TCM acupuncture, or any other style I had witnessed until then.

But an indomitable spirit and unwillingness to back down in the face of difficulties were the primary reasons for her success, in my opinion. Placing the methods she used in the hands of one more timid would not yield the same results.

Of course she was human, the pain she had reduced by eighty percent in the first treatment would come back in a day or two, and chronic complaints or major diseases were "managed" instead of cured, just like with other acupuncturists. But her willingness – insistence really – to give each patient as much relief as possible in each treatment built an incredibly committed and enthusiastic client base.

Over the past few years, I have come to see persistence as one of the most important qualities a person can have in life, an unsung hero that is essential to any meaningful success, and I am grateful to Kiiko for showing me how far simply not giving up can take you.

But underlying these three attributes – communication, inspiration, persistence – is another quality that is perhaps even more essential: confidence. No matter what quality you rely on to foster connections with patients, if they smell fear, they will not be coming back. Without confidence, the treatment plans you present will lack conviction, your attempts to inspire will fall flat and you will not have the spine to surmount obstacles. Unfortunately, trying to build faith in yourself can be a vicious circle: you need confidence to succeed but it is difficult to do a good job without confidence.

Luckily, it seems success is much more powerful than failure. Six bungled treatments will sit heavily on a practitioner, but this feeling is easily lifted by a single satisfied patient. Being told, "Wow, I feel so much better," by just one person can erase the malaise brought on by a string of, "No, not much change." Perhaps this is because failure is investment in success. Setbacks hurt, but there is no better way to figure out what needs to be improved than by seeing your present methods and ideas flop.

It is now about two years since I left Boston and my day-to-day contact with these three practitioners ended. Where am I now? Have I taken these lessons to heart and plowed them into a practice that is now thriving? Unfortunately (or maybe fortunately, who knows in life), the answer is "no." My life took a sharp left turn in late 2009 and I now find myself in Tokyo working for a Japanese newspaper.

Due to a variety of reasons – including probably a lack of persistence on my part – my clinical career is on hold. But when the twists and turns of my life bring me back to the treatment table, I will be a wiser practitioner. I will provide patients clarity in terms of their choices, as much inspiration as I can muster, and will stand firmly beside them in their quests for well-being.

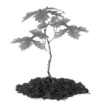